Journey Through Pneumonia

By
Lynne D M Noble

Copyright 2021 Lynne D M Noble

Independently published

Contents

About the Author

Lynne Noble was born in 1953 in Huddersfield, West Yorkshire. From a very early age, Lynne showed an interest in nutrition and genetics avidly reading any books that she could get her hands on at the time.

Initially, Lynne studied orthopaedics but events led her to work with the elderly mentally infirm. Here, her interest in neurodegenerative disorders and pain syndromes developed.

Lynne undertook rigorous programmes of study, completing her Cert Ed., (FE) BSc (Hons) and Adv. Dip Education simultaneously before moving onto her M.Ed.

From there she took further demanding programmes in Human Nutrition, Pharmacology, Neuroscience, Genetics and Immunology. During this time, she was given many prestigious awards for her academic work. It was noted then that Lynne was not afraid of tackling difficult subjects.

She began her law degree but ill health prevented her from pursuing this. However, in this time, she moved from being a foster parent to adoptive parent.

She has been instrumental in setting up projects in the community for disadvantaged groups.

She is a member of the Guild of Health Writers and the British Union of Journalists

Now retired, she lives with her husband in a historic Georgian riverside town in the West Midlands. She enjoys gardening, watching her husband bowling and researching.

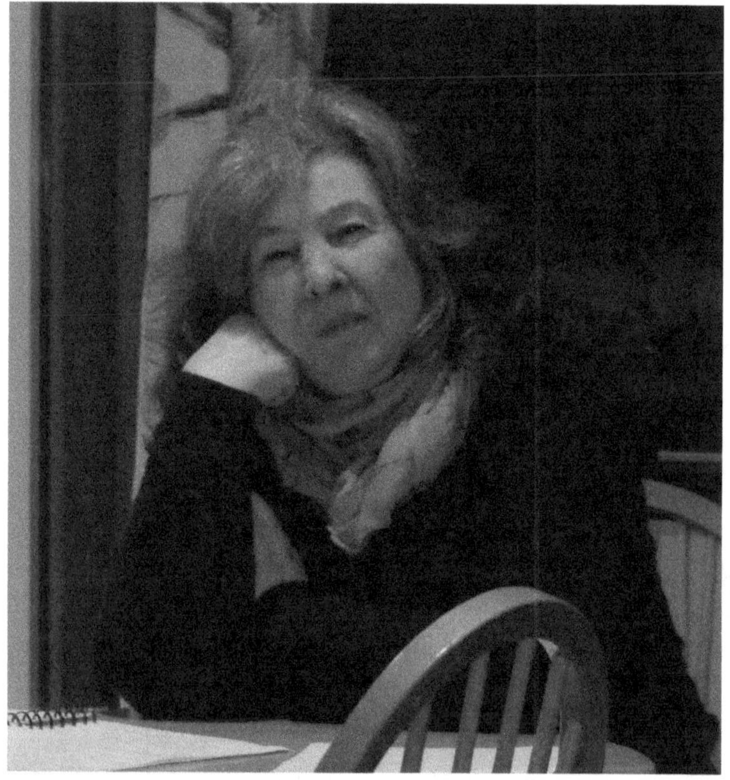

Author Lynne Noble at home

https://quintessentiallylynne.weebly.com/nutritional-medicine.html

Preface

Respiratory conditions run in my husband's family but through good nutrition, warmth and rest, we have managed to get through winter without much harm.

This year,2021, my nearly 76-year-old husband – along with just about everyone else that we knew - contracted a particularly nasty form of pneumonia.

 In elderly people the outcome is not good. Recovery may not be complete and there may be permanent damage to the lungs so there is need for a book to explain not only how to avoid getting pneumonia but also how to address it during and post pneumonia if it does occur.

This is such a book.

It combines the most recent and relevant research with an extensive knowledge of nutrition as a medicine and immunology and infectious disease. However, the experience of caring for a family member with it, softens the approach so that it is relevant and amenable to all.

As always, how illness is addressed - beyond traditional medicine using nutrition as (adjunctive) therapy - will always form the main subject matter of my books. The judicious use of diet and supplements to prevent and treat illness cannot be underplayed.

Thankfully, even if an individual does get pneumonia, most cases are not dealt with in hospital. That experience is what is reserved for the more severe cases. However, with a bit of planning, this book will help show you how to avoid being hospitalised or even succumbing to pneumonia in the first place.

Succumbing to any infectious disease is a gentle warning that there is something amiss in the immune system that needs correcting, sub nutrition is rife and not as visible as the ravages of overt malnutrition.

We have only to consider zinc – a huge player in the immune system – which is used in the synthesis of over 800 macromolecules and 300 enzymes to realise that if we are zinc deficient then an awful lot can go wrong in the body.

The book is intended to show you how to strengthen the immune system through bespoke nutrition so that infection cannot take hold in the first place and, if it should, how to deal with it swiftly.

Types of Pneumonia

Pneumonia is an infection but the underlying infection may be bacterial, viral or fungal in origin. It may infect one lobe in one lung or many lobes in both. It may be patchy -   and will therefore be referred to as bronchopneumonia - and, in this case, it will affect both lungs.

The most common cause of bacterial pneumonia is *Streptococcus Pneumoniae.* Old age, impaired immune systems, underlying conditions and malnutrition, all hasten its ability to infect and spread throughout the lung tissue causing enormous damage in the process.

Bacterial pneumonia will take advantage of those who are weakened after viral infection or who smoke, drink alcohol heavily or have other respiratory diseases such as asthma, COPD or chronic bronchitis.

Viral pneumonia often occurs after a bout of flu but other viruses are involved in initiating this illness, too. Often viral pneumonia will occur initially and, having weakened the body's immune defences, will allow bacterial pneumonia to take hold and flourish. This often necessitates strong antibiotics and steroids if breathing is compromised and the administration of oxygen.

Steroids are counterproductive since they weaken the immune system by depressing the inflammatory processes which are required to take defensive action against infective agents.   Thus these medications – antibiotics and steroids- take over the defensive function of the body, but the latter would work properly if the body was supplied with the proper nutrients it needs to keep the immune system ticking over at optimum performance.   Further, optimum nutrition does not produce the negative side effects that antibiotics and steroids do.

 If viral pneumonia occurs in isolation then the treatment is warmth, rest and small nutritious meals. Viral pneumonia does not respond to antibiotics. It too, can follow other seasonal respiratory viruses which may have temporarily weakened the body's defences.

Mycoplasma Pneumoniae is referred to as atypical pneumonia as the signs and symptoms are dissimilar to viral or bacterial pneumonia. It tends to affect all age groups.

Mycoplasma Pneumoniae (MP) is one worth looking at a little further since it is the one found in community acquired pneumonia; knowing one's enemy MP d goes a long way to defeating it.

MP spreads easily through contact with respiratory fluids. Thus someone sneezing in your vicinity or not washing their hands and touching the same hand rail as you is a great way to spread it

MP damages the lining of the respiratory tract. While it is found mainly in upper respiratory tract   infections with cold and sinusitis like symptoms and - more commonly found as a community acquired infections - it is found in the lower respiratory tract as a pneumonia in 5-10% of cases.

The incubation period for MP is approximately 3 weeks; long enough to forget when you were sneezed over so that you breathe a sigh of relief and think it doesn't matter if you don't take extra vitamin D as a precaution.

However, low adherence proteins are produced and are already beginning to cause damage unbeknown to you. They attach themselves to the epithelial membranes especially in the respiratory tract and produce the chemical hydrogen peroxide and superoxide causing injury to the cell and the tiny little hairs, known as cilia, which waft toxic material away from the lungs. They also produce inflammatory chemicals which, because they can cross react with some cells like red blood cell and neurons produce an auto immune reaction.

The autoimmune response is a risk factor for further related conditions such as transverse myelitis, thrombocytopenia, arthritis, acute hepatitis and others.

Even the organelles are specifically shaped to drive into the cilia producing a sloughing of cell which leads to bouts of prolonged coughing.

As you can see it can make you very ill but much of this is going on without your knowledge for a number of weeks before it suddenly makes its presence known in no uncertain terms.

My husband has only ever had pneumonia once. It was doing its rounds in the complex we were in but as a couple we were fit and well. We had been out shopping one cold winter's day and arrived back home full of energy ready to prepare an early evening meal. We worked together and finally sat down still chatting animatedly. My husband was on the third of his four sausages when he said he could not eat any more. This was a first; it cannot be said that he had anything but a hearty appetite, normally

He did not really know why he felt unwell, the symptoms were vague to begin with until he developed a pain in the right hand side of his chest to the point where he could only get comfortable by sitting forward on a chair and laying his head on a pillow on the table. That's how quickly it can develop.

While there are other pneumonias such as fungal types, the bacterial, viral and mycoplasma are the ones most commonly seen.

Understanding the signs and symptoms of pneumonia can indicate the type it is before other tests confirm it. This is useful given that treatment should be given as soon as possible but even better if we can recognise it for what it is in the community and address it nutritionally so that these infections cannot take hold in the first place.

To this end, a table is supplied below which will help you distinguish them. If symptoms overlap, then it may be that more than one type of infection is present. Remember that they are opportunistic and will take advantage of a weakened system.

Table showing the symptoms of the different types of pneumonia

bacterial	viral	mycoplasma
Green, yellow or bloody phlegm	Follow those of bacterial pneumonia and	Sore throat
Fever, sweating	headache	Fever
Fatigue and confused mental state	Muscle pain	Cough with mucous
Rapid breathing and/or pulse	Feeling weak	
Sharp stabbing pain on coughing or breathing	Worsening of cough	
Shortness of breath		
Bluish colour to fingernails and lips		

Please note that the symptoms in children can present very differently and even in adults, the manifestation of symptoms may differ due to genetic differences.

If you present to your GP with a respiratory tract infection they may order tests to ascertain the type of infection and how it is presenting itself; chest x rays, blood tests and the amount of oxygen present in your blood stream will normally be ordered or determined.

The results of these will shape your treatment plan and how your future needs will be met.

These will be discussed more fully later in the book but may include a bronchoscopy, a CT scan and an echocardiogram.

However, what if we could avoid this altogether; is that not what we should be aiming for? Prevention rather than cure?

Let's take a step back and look at one way of how the immune system may be compromised.

Vitamin C is able to retain immune cell function. Research exists that showed that the elderly who took large doses of vitamin C every day for a year retained a constant number of immune cells. In contrast those who did not had fewer cells and those had less effective function.

We know that many people are vitamin D deficient but a deficiency – or insufficiency – of vitamin C is met with signs of disbelief; this could never happen in a country such as ours…….. only it does for the Recommended Dietary intake (RDI) of 75mg for women and 90mg for men is, in my opinion, far too low and even lower for vulnerable groups like pregnant women or the elderly who eat less and absorb less of the nutrients that they do take in.

 This seems to be a good place to stop for the moment and look at my husband's experience of bacterial pneumonia before re-joining the more formal informative aspects of it later. Information appears to be much more accessible when set down within a patient's experience and offers an oasis from a multitude of dry facts.

The Background

This book came about at a time when my 75-year-old husband – who had always been susceptible to respiratory infections – had a particularly nasty bout of bacterial pneumonia in early 2021.

He has always been prone to bronchitis in winter, due to a hereditary condition, but once the spring heralded, he recovered well and maintained more energy than people ten or fifteen years younger.

We got used to the annoying cough that materialised every December. 'Just a virus,' the Nurse Practitioner had stated breezily. 'Keep warm, drink plenty of fluids and get plenty of rest and you will be fine in three or four weeks.'

And he was. He did not ever need antibiotics although on one occasion he was given an inhaler. However, it remained unused in his drawer.

Of course, as a precautionary measure, he had x-rays. His lungs were clear so that was OK. In all his 75 years he had only had an operation for bunions, minor back problems, after a road traffic accident, and sleep apnoea which we dealt with successfully.

On the rare occasions that we moved house, and he had to attend a GP for an initial consultation, his low blood pressure became a talking point. On every occasion, the medic involved would tap their machine and declare it 'not working' before striding out of the room to find another sphygmometer that would be more accommodating.

On one occasion, a GP did remark that if my husband's blood pressure dropped any lower, then they would have to medicate. As no-one ever followed this up, it never became a problem.

So, whenever the cold weather came, I would instruct my husband to take extra vitamin D and zinc as a precautionary measure to help him through the winter. This appeared to work very well for ten years and we weathered the cold and damp, in the unforgiving climate of West Yorkshire, very well.

 My husband   did not have an aversion to doctors but had been brought up in a pre NHS era and any childhood ailment - not that he can remember having any - was dealt with by rest and Lucozade. He certainly wasn't cossetted and complained bitterly if anything came along that might curtail his activities. Trips to the GP were a rare event for him.

The bacterial pneumonia – which had been going around the community – struck swiftly. My husband

and I had been shopping without any problems. We had arrived back at home at 2.30pm and my husband said that he would make lunch which he did. That was on the table at 3pm.

At that point he did not have any symptoms of pneumonia – no cough, fever, pain or breathlessness.

If there was even the slightest hint that he was unwell it was that he left one of the four sausages he had served himself, uneaten– an unheard of event!

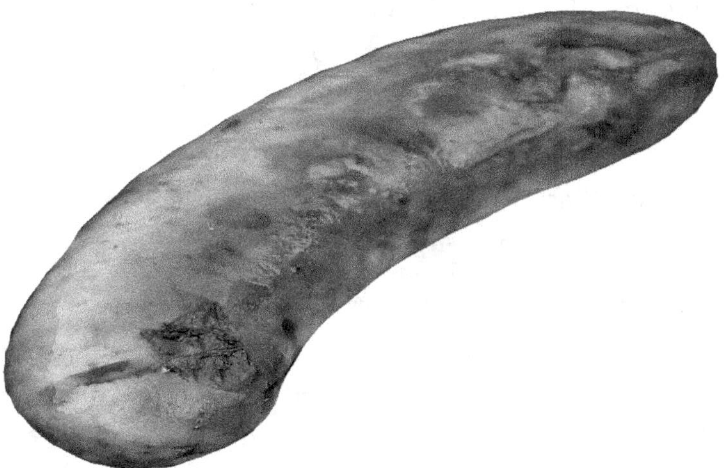

He left a sausage on his plate so I knew he was unwell.

An hour later he said that he felt tired but this was not an unusual occurrence after a meal. He said he felt a little breathless, but would have a nap.

An hour later he woke up. He said he still felt breathless and there was a strange ache in his side for which he took some paracetamol and some ibuprofen.

Shortly after, he started complaining of a stabbing pain in his left side. He could not sit in the armchair nor get into bed due to the pain and had to sit on a dining chair with his head on a pillow while I phoned emergency.

By this time, it was clear he had a temperature. In addition, his SATS which had registered no abnormalities earlier had dropped to 92 (normally 99) and he was tachycardic with a pulse rate of 105 whereas it was normally just under 70 beats per minute.

I also called the care staff that were on duty in the complex that I lived in. They heard all the information that I gave to the emergency team

The emergency department ran through a checklist of questions and decided that my husband did not score enough points to warrant an ambulance – something that I found very strange indeed. I disagreed with them but they said they would pass on this information onto 111 and suggested that he go to his GP the following morning.

I must admit that I was quite angry at this. My husband could not move due to the pain, nor could he get into bed. His condition had worsened dramatically in a very short space of time. It was debatable whether he would be here the following morning. Even if he was, there was no way that I could have got him to the GP.

We ran through the checklist again. I kept repeating that he was tachycardic, had a temperature, was in a lot of pain when he was breathing. The lady I spoke to sounded unconvinced.

'I will have to speak to my supervisor,' she announced.

'I have medical qualifications.' I blurted out.

There was a silence and then. .....

I'm sorry did you say that you had medical qualifications? What are they? What do you do?'

So I told her.

'! think I will do the checklist again,' she muttered. She carried this out – my answers were the same - and this time it was found that my husband **did** qualify for an ambulance.

The ambulance arrived quickly by which time I had written medical details down. When he arrived at hospital he was given a lateral flow test which proved negative as I would expect. He was also given blood tests.

He was placed on steroids, intravenous antibiotics and oxygen. Apparently, he had a severe form of bacterial pneumonia. He was also given antibiotics directly into his abdominal area. He wasn't impressed with that and says he would not have that again.

The two main antibiotics that he was prescribed were Clarithromycin and Co-amoxiclav.

Clarithromycin is a macrolide antibiotic. This means that it has a particular structure. They are bacteriostatic which means that they suppress or inhibit bacterial growth as opposed to killing bacteria outright.

Macrolides are normally used to treat gram positive bacterial infections such as Streptococcus pneumonia but they do have a limited application for some gram negative bacteria.

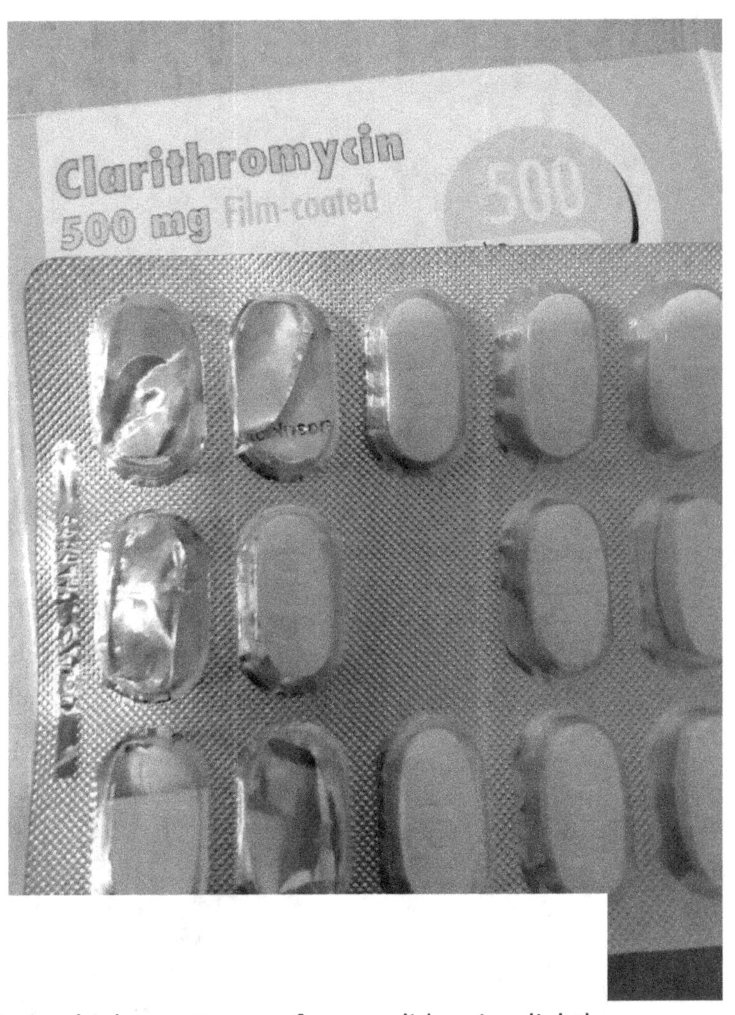

The antimicrobial spectrum of macrolides is slightly wider than penicillin and is therefore a good substitute for those who are allergic to penicillin.

Macrolides can also be administered in a number of ways.

Co-Amoxiclav is a combination of amoxicillin and clavulanic acid. Some bacteria have a chemical defence which they use to outwit the immune system. Clavulanic acid blocks this defence.

 Amoxicillin is a commonly used antibiotic and works by disrupting a bacterium's ability to form cell walls. Thus its function is to destroy rather than inhibit the growth of bacteria.

All in all it was a good cocktail of drugs.

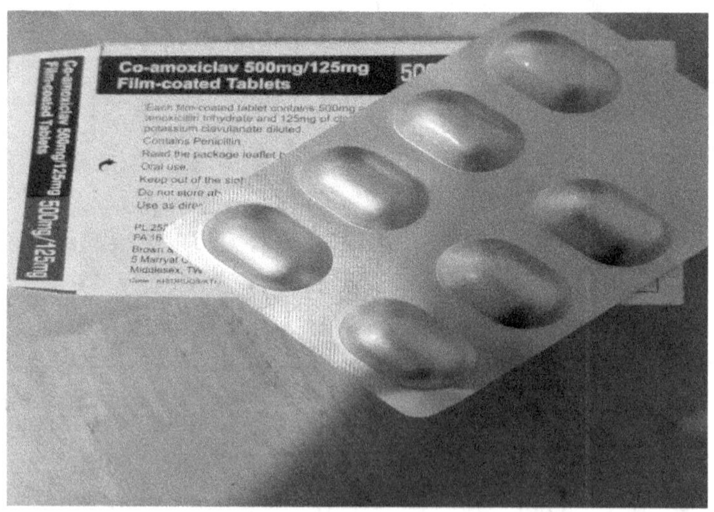

My husband was also placed on blood thinners because there is a tendency for blood to form blood clots in infections such as these. There are a number of blood thinners that can be prescribed. I suggested that he declined Rivaroxaban as there are class actions out against the manufacturers in the US and the UK.

In addition, this medication is well known for causing severe and intractable constipation. When you have pneumonia that is the last thing that you need. It is just adding insult to injury.

In the end my husband plumped for Apixaban and appears to be fine with that. It is a 14-day course after which he had to stop completely.

If I had been allowed to visit it, I would have done things differently but due to world events visiting was not allowed. There was a sense of profound helplessness on my part. For example, numerous studies show the impact of vitamin D deficiency and the increased risk of blood clotting; it may be that those with sufficient levels of vitamin D may not be at risk of abnormal blood clotting and could forego medication with the side effects of the popularly prescribed anti blood clotting medications.

 One study,[1] which appeared in the Post Graduate Medical Journal, showed that there was a significant decrease in fibrinogen on high-dose cholecalciferol supplementation. Cholecalciferol is the active form of vitamin D also known as vitamin D3.

---

[1] https://pmj.bmj.com/content/early/2020/11/12/postgradmedj-2020-139065

Fibrinogen is a protein, a coagulating agent that is vital for blood clot formation. It is synthesised in the liver and released by the liver when it is required.

Fibrinogen is also a biomarker of inflammation so that when levels are elevated it indicates that inflammation is present.

Individuals with a high risk of cardiovascular events can be identified by the presence of high fibrinogen levels.

The participants in the trial were randomised to receive either 60,000 [2]IU's of cholecalciferol (intervention group) or a placebo (control group) for a period of seven days.

Fibronogen markers – amongst others – were measured periodically and were significantly decreased in those with cholecalciferol supplementation.

As vitamin D is also necessary for making an anti-microbial called cathelicidin then it appears to make more sense prescribing vitamin D than the blood thinners that are currently on the market as the latter can have significant adverse effects.

I mention one acquaintance who had been on Rivaroxaban, for a number of years. without any follow up. They began to get numerous haemorrhages in their

---

[2] The recommended daily dosage is in the region of 1000 IU's. This may be too low for those with absorption problems such as Crohn's disease, elderly, those on low fat diets as fat is needed to absorb vitamin D and those with dark skin which protects from some of the sun's rays vital for making vitamin D in the skin.

eyes, followed by bleeding from the bowel and urinary system in quite a dramatic way. Spontaneous bruising also appeared.

Rivaroxaban was stopped and it cleared up completely. The individual is now taking 4,000 IU's of vitamin D daily.

At the end of this book, I will add more details about those who are risk of vitamin D deficiency and its sources.

HICCUPS

A debilitating side effect of my husband's pneumonia was intractable hiccups. This may sound strange and even met with a slight smile at the thought of it. However, my husband was unable to eat, sleep or talk properly because of their constant presence and was, understandably, fatigued by them.

He had had them in the past and had to be medicated with chlorpromazine which did the trick. At the time we were not aware of the familial lung condition he had and we just put it down to a quirk. The usual tricks of clasping your knees to your chest for a couple of minutes, holding your breath and other well-known methods did not work.

The phrenic nerves, which run through the lungs, become irritated during respiratory infections. They are the only nerves that control the diaphragm so are vital to breathing. They make the diaphragm contract but it becomes abnormally so when irritation of these nerves occur. This results in hiccups.

Phrenic nerves originate in the cervical spine, make their way down the length of the neck and through the chest to the diaphragm

Disorders found in the abdomen may result in referred pain in the shoulder due to this phrenic nerve layout.

As it was, my husband's hiccups did not go away. He came home with them and I had to contact the GP to ask for a prescription like the one that he had previously.

These did not work this time and, as we did not know how long it would take for the inflammation, causing irritation of the phrenic nerve to go away, we could not just wait for this symptom to go. I suggested Pregabalin (Lyrica) and this did work very well and immediately. Five days, later as the antibiotics did their job, he found that the hiccups had dissipated and he no longer needed the Pregabalin.

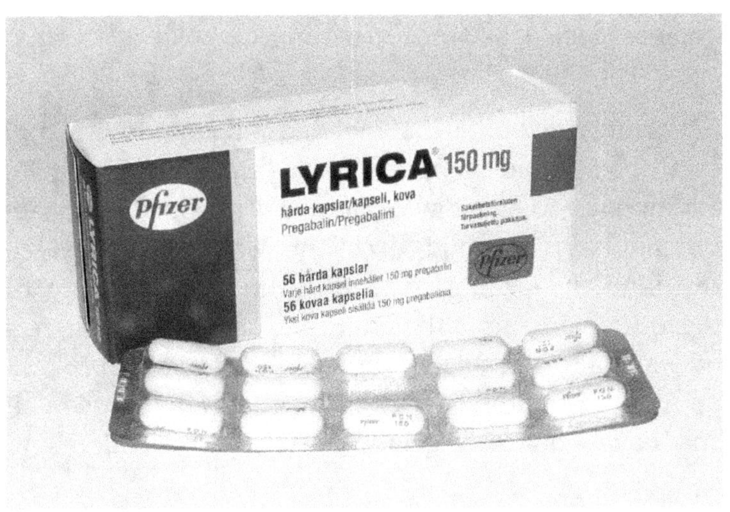

Pregabalin also is used to treat anxiety so is useful in this respect too as having pneumonia can - understandably - cause the patient to be anxious.

As pneumonia can appear in quite a dramatic way - even before observations appear to register the presence of an infection - hiccupping should be taken as a sign that there is something going on especially in those who are susceptible to respiratory infection.

Most of us will get hiccups in our lives at some point but that does not mean it is normal to do so if they go beyond more than a short time.

Phrenic nerves become irritated for a reason.

At the time, my husband and I had only recently moved to this address. My nutritional medicine cupboard was depleted and I had not had time to build it back up again.

However, vitamin B1 (300mg) and magnesium (300mg) calm the phrenic nerve very well – and work rapidly. In addition, up to 6g a day of vitamin C needs to be taken. Vitamin C is beyond excellent when it comes to restoring damaged tissue. Of course, the beauty of these supplements is that you can keep them in; there's no waiting to see a doctor or having to travel out to pick up a prescription; just make sure that if you move you still have your medicine cupboard fully loaded and complete.

Diagram showing left phrenic nerve

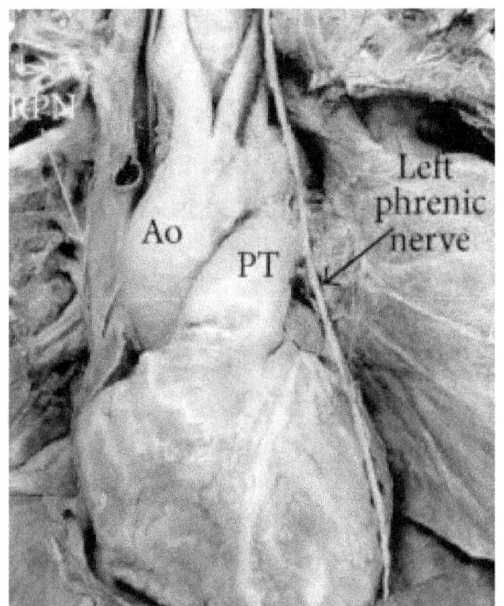

Phrenic Nerve Cadaver

Pleural effusion and adjacent consolidation

Pleural effusion is commonly referred to as 'water on the lungs. It can be one of the more troubling symptoms because as soon as you try to lie down you cannot breathe. It feels like you are drowning and, in my husband's case,It also brought hiccups on with a vengeance.

The fluid builds up in a specific place between the layers of the pleura which are the membranes that enclose the lungs and chest cavity Their function is to lubricate and aid breathing.

Most of the time my people cannot not catch their breath even when well propped up with pillows. It tends to be most comfortable sitting on a dining chair with a pillow or two on the table. Many people prefer to sleep like this for a couple of nights with the quilt wrapped around them.

The main symptoms of pleural effusion are:

- Pain
- Dry cough
- Feeling of chest heaviness/tightness
- Fatigue
- Inability to lie flat
- Inability to exercise
- A feeling of general unwellness (not surprisingly).

Consolidation means that the air which normally occupies the small airways in your lungs is replaced with something else. These can be:

- The products of infection such as phlegm
- A blood clot
- A tumour

The symptoms of consolidation include:

1. coughing up blood or green sputum
2. rapid breathing
3. A dry cough
4. Noisy breathing
5. Fever
6. Fatigue
7. Chest pain and heaviness

Patients may not have all the symptoms.

Consolidation adjacent to the pleural effusion could be due to the pneumonia but questions may be raised if there is a hilar enlargement. Thus, the possibility of malignancy needed to be considered which may have contributed to the weakened state.

The hilar lobe

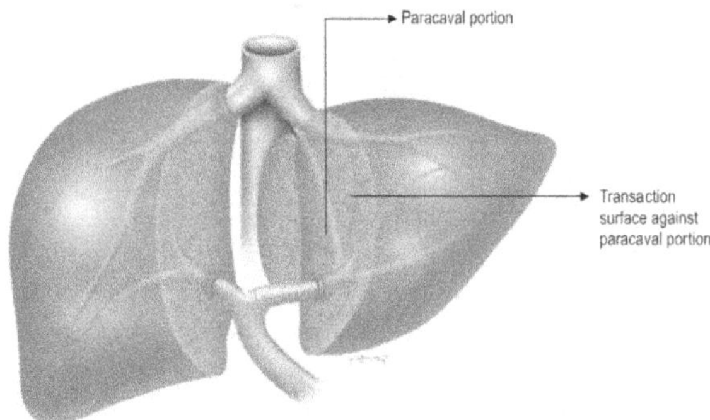

Figure 2 - Anterior approach after opening the interlobar plane and exposing the anterior surface of the paracaval portion and the hilar plate. The paracaval portion is detached from the hilar plate

The hilar lobe is found at the area that attaches the lung root to the main part of the lung.

This was an area away from the main site of the infection.

As the enlargement of the hilar lobe was unilateral, then consideration of the differences found in bilateral and unilateral enlargement were made. This is a useful exercise to eliminate potential causes.

These can be found in the table below.

Potential causes of unilateral and bilateral hilar enlargement

Unilateral	Bilateral
Infection – TB, viral, bacterial	Sarcoidosis/silicosis
Tumour – lung cancer or lymphoma Metastases of lung head/neck, thyroid or testes	Infection – TB, viral, bacterial
Vascular – pulmonary arterial aneurysm/stenosis	Tumour -lymphoma -metastases
	Vascular – pulmonary hypertension COPD – mitral valve disease -left to right shunt - recurrent embolism

On the unilateral side of the table the likely cause of the enlarged hilar lobe are in order that they are presented in the table.

Pulmonary arterial hypertension may be present. This condition is generally referred to in notes as PAH. In this condition the very small arteries in the lungs are either blocked or narrowed. As such it is much harder for blood to flow through them. The blood pressure becomes raised and the heart has to work harder to get it throw those tiny arteries.

The inflammatory processes involved in infectious disease are generally the cause of such blockages. The immune system is very efficient when it detects an infectious agent, sometimes too efficient. PAH should resolve but in some cases doesn't.

This scenario does weaken the heart muscles and, as a result, heart failure may occur.

Heart failure is the inability of the heart to be able to keep up with the body's demands.

The blocking and narrowing of the pulmonary arteries can occur for all sorts of reasons. These include:

- Infection
- Blood clots in the lungs
- Autoimmune diseases
- Heart defects
- Lung disease like bronchitis
- HIV

- Sleep apnoea
- Liver malfunction such as cirrhosis of the liver

Sleep apnoea appears to be very much linked to those who are overweight although I have known quite thin people suffer from this, too. While losing weight does help some people, it does not help everyone. Singing may strengthen the flabby muscles which appear to contribute to it. Further, vitamin C is an excellent anti-inflammatory and may be useful in those who appear to have some form of chronic inflammatory upper respiratory tract condition so that mouth breathing becomes the norm.

Sometimes, symptoms of chest pain, fainting and fatigue may manifest; breathlessness may be evident when walking up a hill that may present no problem for others. PAH may appear to come and go and, in some cases, only swelling of the right leg may indicate its presence as the heart struggles with what it has to do.

PAH is generally a progressive disease although treating infection or blood clots may alleviate the condition by removing the blockage or reducing the narrowing. The increase in limb size is a good indicator of how well the heart is coping with current events.

Most of the time there is hardly any difference in limb size and the PAH appears to have stabilised; one notable difference was when my husband and I were on holiday and for some inexplicable reason, his right leg swelled so much that he was unable to put his shoes and socks on. To this day we have no idea of the cause but it has not happened again.

When the heart appears to be struggling then medics tend to use diuretics to remove the excess fluid. Trust us to be on holiday on a cruise ship when my husband's leg swelled up to the extent that it did. We did have vitamin C and magnesium which both have diuretic effect and these appeared to do the trick.

Where would we be without vitamin C and magnesium?

Scarring of lung tissue tends to occur. When scarring occurs the lung tissue becomes thickened and stiffer. This makes the transference of oxygen from the lungs into the bloodstream difficult and organs and the brain may suffer as a result. People with pneumonia can become confused very easily.

Scarring may also increase the risk of lung cancer. It is therefore of the utmost importance that pneumonia is never allowed to gain hold.

Even when intravenous antibiotics followed by an oral course are completed the infection may still not be resolved although the patient, looking bright and reasonably alert enough to be sent home, feels well enough to go home and is discharged. Although it is uncommon breathlessness may occur and if a stethoscope is placed in the appropriate position then crackles may be heard. The stabbing pain typical of pneumonia may follow so on discharge, and in order to avoid this, therapeutic doses of vitamin c and vitamin D in the order of 6g of vitamin c and 10,000 IUs' of vitamin D should be given daily along with 300mg magnesium and 50mg zinc.

Zinc is needed to build up tissue and pneumonia destroys lung tissue providing even more ways for infection to take hold.

We will look at these nutrients in more detail in the next chapter for, while undoubtedly, measures such as antibiotics, steroids and oxygen all aid recovery, these are all measures which are implemented by the doctor and it is becoming increasingly difficult to find one at times. Time is of the essence when it comes to pneumonia; we can't sit and wait around. Further, antibiotic resistance is a real thing but bespoke nutrition has always been the body's preferred source of healing. We just need to understand what does what so that we can begin treatment until further help arrives or continue it if no help arrives.

It is to this subject that we shall turn to next.

Vitamin D – immune system regulator

Vitamin D is one of the unsung heroes of the vitamin world. When people think about vitamin D – if they do at all - they think of it in association with healthy bones. Most people do not realise that vitamin D makes its own broad spectrum antimicrobial called cathelicidin. Further, as the majority of the world are vitamin D deficient, this suggests that the majority of the world aren't harnessing the power contained within their own immune systems so that we are becoming increasingly reliant on external forms of treatment which often are not as effective and can carry serious side effects.

An antimicrobial is an agent that kills microorganisms or stops their growth. Cathelicidin consists of small antimicrobial peptides. They are part of our innate immune system and show a broad spectrum of antimicrobial activity against

- Bacteria
- Enveloped viruses
- Fungi

As well as exerting direct antimicrobial effects such as punching holes in the cell membranes of invaders, cathelicidin can also trigger specific defence responses in the host.

Vitamin D upregulates the production of cathelicidin and is found to exert an effect in many organs and systems of the body. This is not surprising since vitamin D receptors can be found throughout the body which evidences the importance it has for human health.

Cathelicidin has been found in the:

- Stomach
- Trachea
- Skin
- Muscle
- Heart
- Kidney
- Lung
- Brain
- Intestine

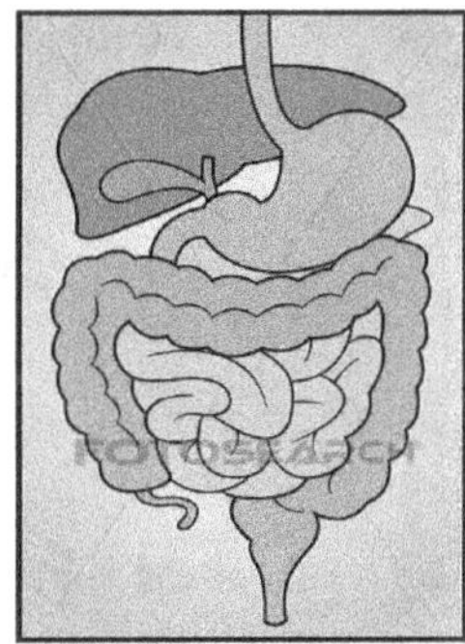

Cathelicidin has been found in the digestive system.

Human cathelicidin acts in the promotion of wound healing and can modulate the adaptive immune system.

It's importance to tissue healing - in the case of pneumonia damaged lung tissue - can be understood.

Higher plasma levels of human cathelicidin antimicrobial protein, which are upregulated by vitamin D, appear to significantly reduce the risk of death from infection in dialysis patients. Studies show that patients with a high level of this protein were 3.7 times more likely to survive kidney dialysis for a year without a fatal infection. This shows how powerful this natural antimicrobial is.

As people get older they are less likely to be able to absorb vitamin D through the action of the sun's rays on their skin. Cholesterol is needed to synthesise vitamin D from the sun so those on statins may not be making as much vitamin D as they thought when sitting out on a sunny day.

Older people and those with inflammatory bowel disease have greater difficulty absorbing any nutrient from food. Further, it is extremely difficult, if not impossible, to obtain sufficient vitamin D from the diet.

Sometimes, elderly people are given prescribed vitamin D supplements but these come in a dry chalky tablet form. If they are not take with a little fat or oil, then the vitamin D simply cannot be absorbed for use by the body. I have never known of anyone prescribed these supplements being given that information.

Vitamin D also needs magnesium for its activation if it is the commonly prescribed inactive form, vitamin D2 as opposed to the active form vitamin D3.

The best sources of vitamin D are oily fish, fortified cereals and eggs. However, you would need to eat 80 eggs daily to obtain sufficient vitamin D for the day. The recommended daily amount is 1000-4000 IU's.

However, as we have already learned in the study, on a short term basis, the amount of vitamin D can be increased significantly providing greater therapeutic benefit. Nevertheless, those on blood thinners need to take advice on how to do this safely given that vitamin D decreases the amount of the blood clotting fibrinogen.

Supplements are advised for

- The elderly
- Those who are housebound
- Those who work indoors
- Those with black skin
- Those on low fat diets
- Those on mainly plant based diets

- Those on some medications. Like cholesterol reducing drugs.
- Those with inflammatory bowel disease or other conditions where the ability to absorb nutrients is compromised.

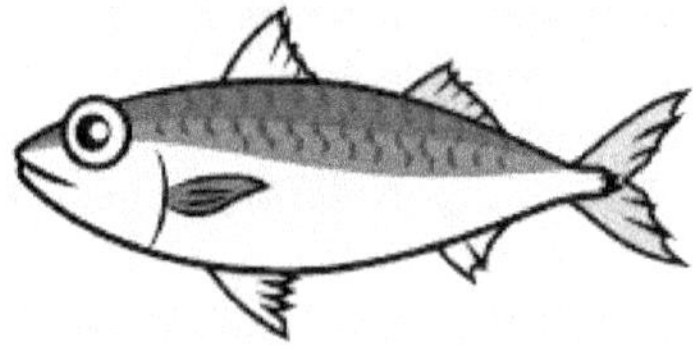

Oily fish such as mackerel, salmon and fresh tuna contain good amounts of vitamin D.

I also do not recommend using omega 6 vegetable oils such as sunflower oils during periods of illness. This is because omega 6 poly unsaturated fatty acids increase inflammation and there is enough going on at the time without adding to it.

Lard is a stable fat and will not increase inflammation. Vitamin D is actually stored in lard so it provides further beneficial nutrients when used in cooking.

Most people who use omega 6 vegetable oils as part of their diet have a tendency to unhealthy and lined skin. Those who use lard and butter – natural fats – have wonderfully smooth and unlined skin.

It would be preferable if people were automatically tested for vitamin D status around September so any deficiency could be corrected before the winter.

When deficiency is found it can accompany lethargy and deep bone pain which is very distressing.

Some people appear to be non-responders to vitamin D supplementation although this corrects itself if 6mg of boron (found in fruit and vegetables) is taken daily. However, most vitamin D cannot be absorbed due to lack of fat in the diet when taken or it cannot be activated due to the lack of magnesium. Nutrients do not exist and function in isolation from others which is why a diverse, nutrient dense diet is the best medicine that you can get.

Quercetin and allicin

Quercetin is a natural pigment or flavonoid which is found in many fruits, vegetables and grains as well as wine and tea. Red onions are particularly rich in quercetin. It has antioxidant properties and these properties help combat the damaging effects of free radicals.

Free radicals are unpaired electrons. These free radicals are the cause of chronic disease which is so rife in society. Antioxidants are able to bind to free radicals and neutralise them in the process. This stops the chronic inflammatory processes which are associated with many diseases including diabetes, lymphoedema, lipoedema, arthritis, high blood pressure, neurodegenerative disorders as well as respiratory conditions like pneumonia. This is not a definitive list.

Quercetin's benefits do not stop there though. It has anti-tumour activity. Its properties inhibit the proliferation of cancer cells by inducing apoptosis (cell death) as well as arresting the cell cycle of cancers. Thus, in matters of lung cancer relating to scarring of lung tissue, quercetin has many benefits.

If this wasn't enough, quercetin has anti-fibrotic activity and is particularly useful to reduce the implications of scarring of lung tissue.

Quercetin is also able to inhibit RNA polymerase, necessary for viral replication.

Given that quercetin is able to reduce inflammation and alleviate many of the other symptoms of pneumonia it is recommended that quercetin on a daily basis is taken at 500mg daily during active infection.

Quercetin is found in good amounts in onion and apple and as these are core soup ingredients then it does not take much imagination to provide a healthy bespoke liquid meal. However, quercetin is an adjuvant. It can be used alongside vitamin D and other more robust treatments but should not be used as the sole treatment.

Allicin is found in garlic and other members of the onion family. It is able to pass through the phospholipid membranes and inhibit viral replication. Img of allicin is also considered to have the equivalent efficacy of 15 IU's of penicillin but with efficacy against gram positive and gram negative bacteria. There is not however a great deal of research on how effective is it against mycoplasma but it will address other opportunistic infections such as Staphylococcus aureus, Salmonella typhi and Listeria monocytogenes which may occur concomitantly.

Raw garlic is better as much of the active ingredient is destroyed when dried.

Zinc

Zinc is a trace element which is often associated with the health of the immune system. Indeed, a zinc deficiency can lead to a vulnerability to infection. Zinc is better known for its ability to activate T lymphocytes. It also has a regulatory role in controlling the immune response as well as attacking cancerous and infected cells. Zinc supplementation studies in the elderly have shown a reduction in the rate   and severity of infections, decreased oxidative stress and the presence of fewer inflammatory cytokines.   However, its super status is not just confined to the health of the immune system.

Zinc is required for many functions in the body especially in relation to activating enzymes which speed up metabolic processes in the body. Some of these processes may be related to wound healing and age-related chronic diseases.

Oxidative stress underlies the molecular mechanisms responsible for the development of many inflammatory diseases The cellular antioxidant system proves insufficient to remove the reactive oxygen species which damage cells and create inflammation in this process.

The regulatory function of zinc cannot be underestimated. It is essential to the structure and function of nearly 800 macromolecules and over 300 enzymes.

Macromolecules are very large molecules such as proteins made from amino acids.

Common macromolecules, monomers and some end products are:

MACROMOLECULE	MONOMERS (the building blocks)	END PRODUCT
protein	Amino acids	Protein – many types such as keratin for hair and collagen for connective tissue, enzymes and **antibodies.**
Nucleic acids	Nucleotides	RNA and DNA
Lipids	Fatty acids	Fats, sterols, waxes and oils

Although Zinc is known for its antiviral impact, it also has a beneficial effect on secretory molecules and the bactericidal activity of human peptidoglycan recognition proteins. (PGLYRP's)

Peptidoglycan is a substance that forms the cell walls of bacteria. The ability of the immune system to detect bacteria – and thus deal with it – is partially dependent on the available serum zinc.

The importance of having adequate daily amounts of zinc cannot be underestimated. Zinc has been described as the element with a minor plasma pool and a rapid turnover. That means it has limited storage capacity in the body and must be taken regularly in food.

There are certain groups of individuals that are more susceptible to zinc deficiency. These include:

- Diabetics
- Cancer patients
- Those with liver disease
- Those on a high plant diet as the phytates in plants bind to zinc
- Those on high copper or high iron diets
- Those who are on a calorie reducing diet
- Those who are under stress
- The elderly
- Breast fed babies
- Pregnant women
- Alcoholism
- Those with malabsorption problems of the digestive tract such as Crohn's disease.

Sources of zinc include:

- Oysters (very high in zinc) 3 ounces provides 673% of the daily value
- Beef – 3 ounces provide 65% of your daily requirements
- Beef patty – 3 ounces provides 64% of your daily requirement
- Baked beans – half a cup provides 26% of your daily requirement.

The Daily Requirement of Zinc has been placed at'

Men – 11g

Women 8mg

However, for short periods of no greater than a month, upwards of this amount may be used to combat bacteria. Indeed, the recommended daily intakes do not appear to be sufficient for the vulnerable groups mentioned.

At the first sign of a bacterial infection 75 -100mg over the course of the day may be taken for 3 days and then reduced to 25mg for the rest of the month until the infection is dealt with.

If you take high dose zinc for much longer you raise the risk of iron and copper depletion which carry their own risk of deficiency diseases some of which will impact the ability of the immune system to do its job properly.

Copper is also required to combat bacteria but any supplementation should be taken at the opposite end of the day to that of zinc.

People suffering from iron deficiency anaemia are also more susceptible to infection as it is required for normal immune system functioning. The bacteriacidal activity of macrophages depends on iron as it is a component of peroxide which macrophages like to drop onto infective agents in order to kill them.

T cells, a vital part of the acquired immune system which is the more specialist response, is also dependent on iron for its function yet groups like the elderly, menstruating age women, pregnant women and those on plant based diets are vulnerable to a deficiency. Unfortunately, there is downside to iron since pathogens also need it for their function. This may be the reason why a little bloodletting was so effective in the olden days.

It is easy for iron deficiency anaemia to be detected through a simple blood test but in its absence simply pull down your lower eyelid gently. There should be evident a rich red network of blood vessels; if white, lemon or peachy in colour then iron deficiency is likely and needs to be corrected as soon as possible in order to keep healthy immune system defences.

I will return to copper and cover it in more detail later.

Co-enzyme Q10

This enzyme is depleted in statin takers and insufficiency occurs during the ageing process, yet it is a powerful antioxidant and reduces the risks of blood clots which are more likely to occur during bouts of pneumonia.

Coenzyme Q10 is required for the synthesis of collagen and elastin. If scarring of tissue has occurred during infection, then co-enzyme Q10 may help ameliorate some of the damage and symptoms caused at the time.

Good sources of co-enzyme Q10 are organ meats like liver, kidney and heart which are also rich in iron. Some muscle meats like chicken and pork contain smaller amounts. Legumes, broccoli, cauliflower and spinach are also good sources of this enzyme.

Inflammation

Just what is inflammation? That's probably a good question for many people. We have an idea when we see redness and swelling that inflammation is going on which will always be accompanied by pain. This pain can be diffuse especially when the source is inflammation occurring internally. The pain may also be referred pain so that it appears elsewhere than the original area of injury.

Researchers at the Medical College of Georgia discovered a nerve centre in a cell layer in the spleen that controls the immune response and therefore inflammation throughout the body. It is quelled by taking 2g of baking soda in water for two weeks.

The only downside to this is that baking soda has the potential to raise your blood pressure. If you do have raised blood pressure, then taking 250mg of magnesium and a glass of tomato juice for the potassium will most likely address this propensity to raised blood pressure. Vitamin C has the ability to lower blood pressure too.

<u>Table showing some of the main differences in the innate immune system and the adaptive/acquired immune system.</u>

Innate immune system	Adaptive immune system
Responds quickly to invaders	Is slower to respond
Has a non-selective action	Is specific in action. eg one white blood cell will react to one specific invader only
Does not make memory cells	Has a long memory for invaders it has already come across.
Composed of a number of defensive reflex actions and substances eg the cough reflex or mucus which is used to trap invaders	Composed of white blood cells and antibodies

Vitamin D specifically enhances the strength of innate and acquired immune system

Medium Chain Fatty Acids

Medium chain fatty acids (MCFA's) are chains of fatty acids which are 6-12 chains long. Due to their length they have special properties. They can be used directly by the liver as a source of energy or they can be changed into ketones. Ketones are substances which the liver produces when it breaks down large amounts of fat for energy.

Ketones can cross the blood brain barrier and be used as fuel instead of glucose which the brain normally uses.

MCFA's are less likely to be turned into fat as they can so easily be turned into energy for immediate use.

Just from this perspective they can be an immediate source of energy when you are ill.

The main sources of MCFA's can be seen in the table below.

Type of MCFA	Source of MCFA's
C6 – caproic acid(hexanoic acid)	butter
C8 – caprylic acid (octanoic acid)	Coconut oil, palm kernel oil, goat cheese, butter
C10 – capric acid – (decanoic acid)	Coconut oil, palm kernel oil
C12 – Lauric acid – (dodecanoic acid)	Coconut oil

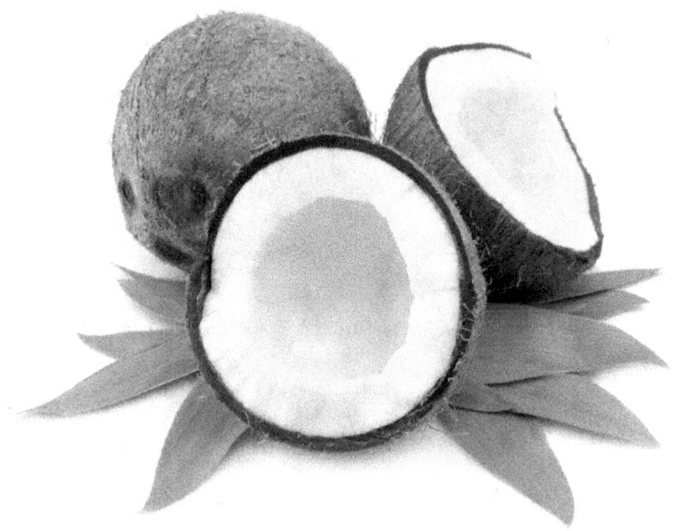

Coconut oil has antibacterial, antifungal, antiviral and antiprotozoal actions in the body. It has unique fatty acids Breast milk contains MCFA's. These help protect the baby when its own immune system is hardly developed.

Studies have shown that MCFA's are effective against viruses causing measles, influenza, pneumonia, throat infections, herpes and AIDS. MCFA'S also are effective against bacteria causing pneumonia, throat infections, stomach infections, sinusitis, rheumatic fever, urinary tract infections, meningitis and dental cavities.

MCFA's are also effective against many fungal infections including those which cause thrush.

While coconut oil is effective against the flu virus, it is not effective against rhinovirus which is one of the viruses which cause the common cold. The MCFA's act on the lipid coating or envelope of the flu virus but the cold virus is not enveloped in a lipid coating.

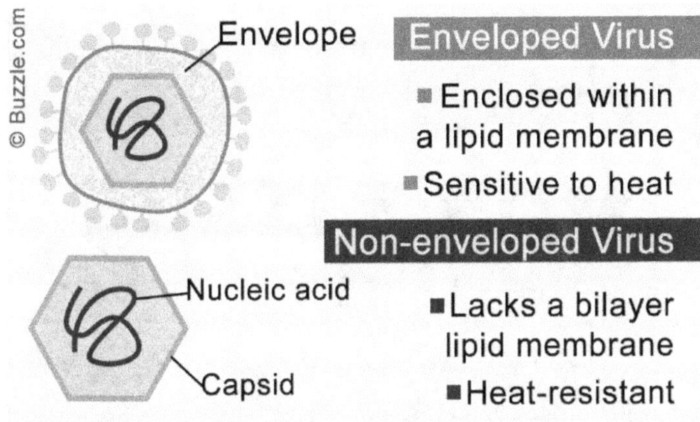

There are many lipid coated viruses and bacteria and these include:

3

Lipid coated viruses
HIV Hepatitis C Measles Herpes simplex Herpes viridae Sarcoma Synctical virus Human lymphotropic virus Vesicular stomatitis virus Visna virus Cytomegalovirus Epstein-Barr virus Influenza Leukaemia virus

---

3 The healing miracle of coconut oil, Bruce Fife N. D pg 61

Pneumonovirus

Lipid coated bacteria
Listeria monocytogenes
Helicobacter pylori
Streptococcus agalactiae
Groups A, B. F & G streptococci
Gram positive organisms
Hemophilus influenza
Staphylococcus aureus

The recommended dosage of coconut oil during illness is 4-8 tablespoonsful daily. This can be stirred into fruit juice to make It more palatable if this is preferred.

A viral infection often precedes bacterial pneumonia by weakening the body's defences to controlling viruses is just as important as addressing the weak points in the body's immune system defences.

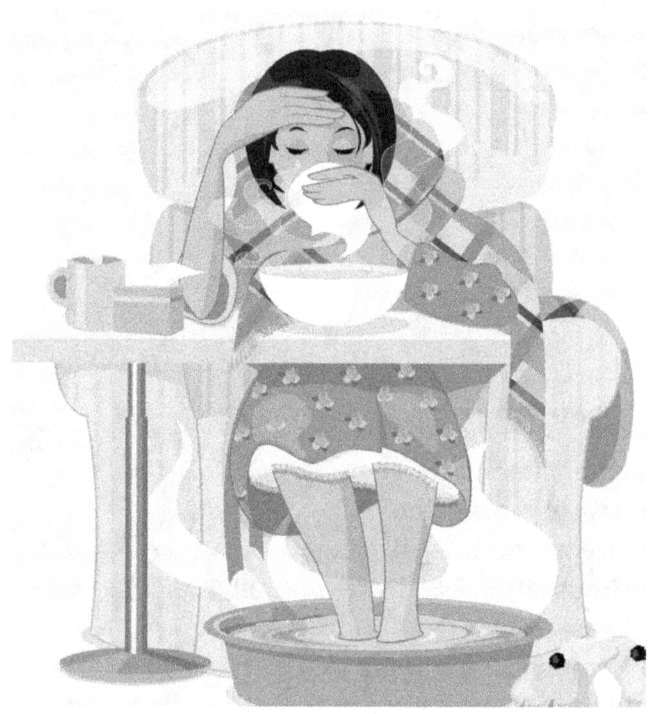

⁴ Studies have shown that coconut oil is effective against the flu virus which may weaken the immune system defences before bacterial pneumonia takes hold.

Curcumin

Curcumin is a natural component of the rhizome *Curcuma Longa* that is also known as turmeric. It is the popular yellow spice which is commonly used in Asian

---

⁴ https://pngtree.com/freepng/influenza-virus-infection_3097745.html

countries in cooking and for medicinal uses. In particular, it is used to treat inflammatory conditions. However, it has also been used to treat diabetes and various types of cancer.

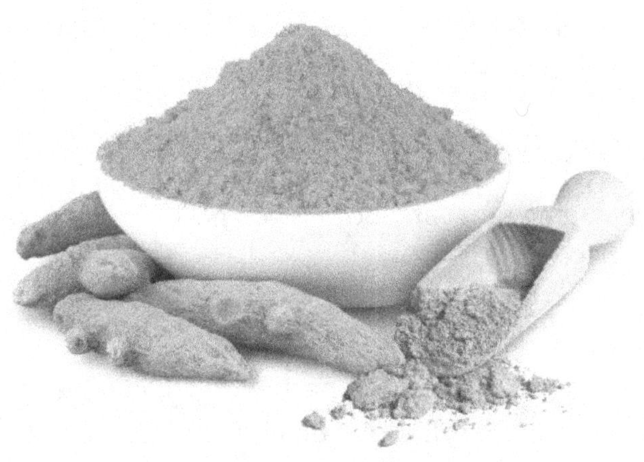

Curcumin has multiple effects and interacts with multiple targets that are involved in inflammation. These include:

- Interleukins
- Tumour necrosis factor

---

5 https://www.indiamart.com/proddetail/pure-turmeric-powder-16143372297.html

Interleukins (IL) are a group of naturally occurring proteins that bring about communication between cells. They regulate cell growth, differentiation and motility. They help stimulate immune responses such as inflammation, helping direct the battle against infection.

Tumour necrosis factor is another cell signalling protein which is involved in the acute inflammatory stage of an infection.

In vitro curcumin has been shown to possess in vitro antimicrobial action against a diversity of infectious agents including fungi and both Gram positive and Gram negative bacteria.

Phenolic compounds

Carvacrol has numerous properties including being a natural antibiotic, an antimicrobial in general, an anti-inflammatory and analgesic.

Carvacrol is a substance found in aromatic plants like oregano, thyme and wild bergamot. It is mildly acidic.

There are a number of foods which contain free and bound phenolic compounds of which carvacrol is one.

Bound phenolic compounds are especially found in cereals. They are important antioxidants. In addition, they inhibit cancerous cell growth and impact on important enzymes which are involved in the metabolism of carbohydrates.

Both free and bound phenols are found in foods such as:

- Peanuts
- Oranges, apples, bananas, red grapes, tomatoes and other highly coloured fruits
- Cocoa
- Milk

Salicylates which are found in aspirin (as a non-food substance) also contain phenols.

There are many other phenolic compounds which contribute to a good strong immune system, Plants sources of phenolic compounds are also known as phytonutrients.

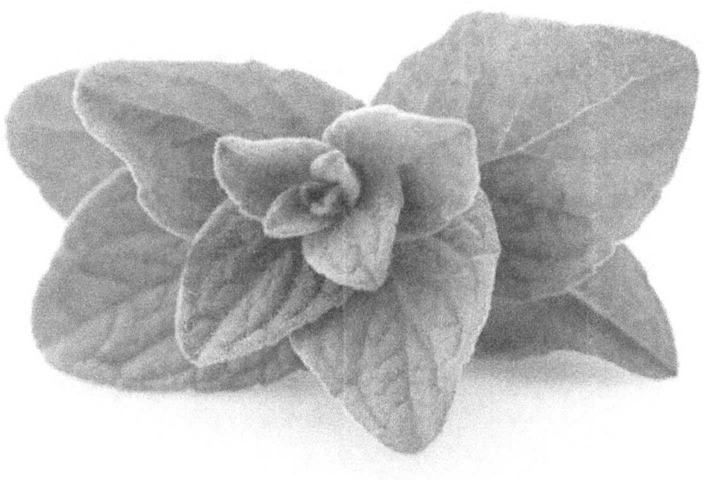

Oregano is a great source of carvacrol

Table showing examples of phytonutrients and their food sources.

Phytonutrient	Food sources
Flavonoids like quercetin and anthocyanins	Soybeans, onions, apples, tea, coffee
Carotenoids like lycopene, lutein, beta carotene, zeaxanthin	Found in orange, red and dark green foods like carrots, tomatoes and dark green leafy veg
Polyphenols like resveratrol and ellagic acid	Red grapes and wine, berries, green tea and whole grains
tannins	Cereals, beans nuts, wine cocoa
curcuminoids	Curcumin from turmeric
Carvacrol	Oregano, thyme, wild bergamot

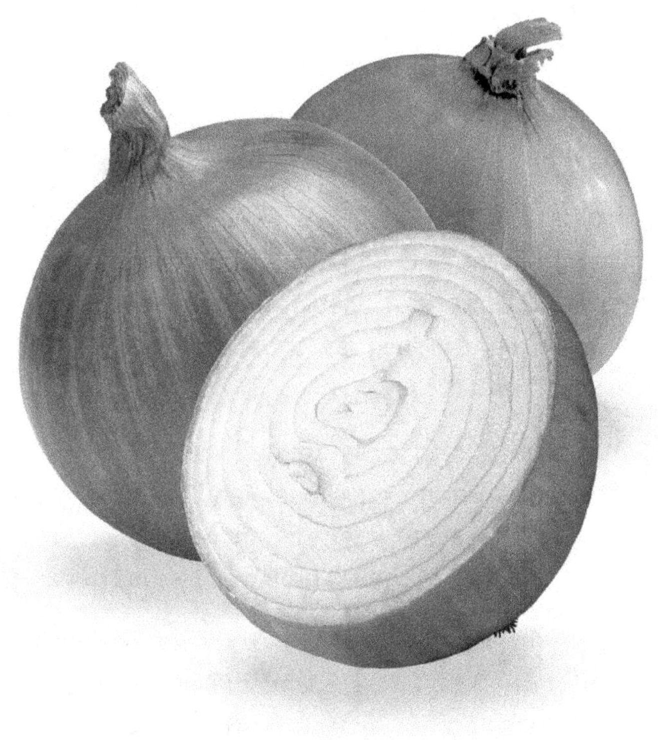

Onions have great anti-inflammatory action

Vitamin C

Early literature has associated vitamin C deficiency with pneumonia and, after this was identified, studies investigated this.

In all nearly 150 animal studies were carried out on diverse infections and findings indicated that vitamin C may prevent or at least alleviate infections caused by a number of agents such as those caused by viruses, bacteria and protozoa.

However, the impact of vitamin C appears to be dose dependent – which makes sense – and the dose used far higher than the recommended daily allowance which is a meagre 75mg for women and 90mg for men.

In these studies, a therapeutic response was not obtained until given at 6-8 grams daily. This represents a huge increase on our expectations of what we require to keep infectious diseases like pneumonia away.

Three controlled trials[6] found that vitamin C prevented pneumonia. Another two controlled trials also found

---

6

https://www.ncbi.nlm.nih.gov/pmc/articles/PMC5409678/#:~:text=In%20the%20ea rly%20literature%2C%20vitamin,bacteria%2C%20viruses%2C%20and%20protozoa.

that treatment with vitamin C benefitted those with pneumonia.

The recommendation then, is that during non-pneumonia times, 1 gram is taking daily in food or through supplementing.

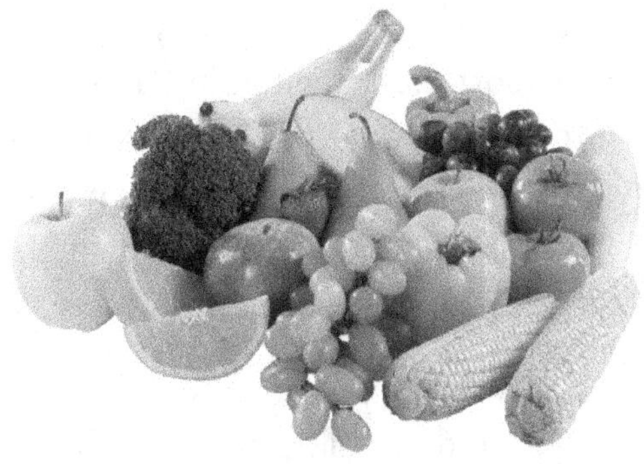

At times when respiratory infection occurs then 8g of vitamin C can be taken daily. This can be frontloaded by 4g initially and then 6 hourly at 1 gm intervals.

Vitamin C is not stored in the body so any excess will simply be eliminated by the kidneys.

How does vitamin C exert its magic? Vitamin C is an antioxidant and thus most beneficial at times of increased oxidative stress.

Many infections activate phagocytes –   these are Pacman - like in their ability to eat up debris – but they also release substances which are known as reactive oxygen species (ROS).

ROS's are damaging to host cells and appear to be involved in the development of infections. The judicious ingestion of vitamin C would go a long way to preventing this.

Phagocytes aid the transportation of vitamin C into cells where it converts into a reduced form. Studies found that when an individual had influenza A infection then the concentration of vitamin C was decreased in the Broncho alveolar lavage fluid with a resultant increase in the oxidised form.

Broncho alveolar lavage fluid is collected after fluid is squirted into a small area of the lung and then collected for analysis. It may contain sputum which is a combination of phlegm and saliva although mucus which had been ejected from the respiratory tract may also be found.

Studies also highlighted that vitamin C deficiency resulted in greater lung disease. Bacterial toxins also decrease the availability of vitamin C to many tissues including lung tissue, studies have found. Indeed, the concentration of vitamin C is found to be ten times higher in the white blood cells of the immune system than in blood plasma, supporting the importance of this vitamin in responding to infection.

Heavy physical stress has been found to affect vitamin C levels because such work increases the amount of ROS in the body as does the presence of infection. Thus to state that only 30mg of vitamin C is required daily for health is a poor assumption.

The RDA of 30mg was set as that was the amount to avoid scurvy not to maintain optimum health. In the same way the RDA for vitamin D was set at a measly 400 IU's which was just enough to prevent rickets but not to maintain optimum health.

When looking at the RDA of any nutrient, it is always wise to ask yourself, 'Why was the RDA set at this level?'

The importance of good nutrition in not only avoiding - but treating - infections such as pneumonia cannot be underestimated.

While we are on the right track by realising that vitamin C and D - among other nutritional substances – undoubtedly play a part in the prevention of respiratory infection, the population do not appear to have grasped that the miniscule amounts recommended by medical establishments do not even begin to therapeutically scratch the surface of the infection.

In addition, vitamin C prevents the replication of viruses and aids maturation of specific immune system cells known as T lymphocytes which are important in dealing with virus. It also assists in the production of interferon.

Interferons are a specific group of proteins released by host cells in response to a number of viruses. The host cells have become infected and will signal – using these proteins - to adjacent cells to increase their defences against viruses.

Isn't the body a wonderful piece of complex machinery?

Vitamin C is easily destroyed by heat and sunlight and storage so foods containing vitamin C should be fresh and eaten as soon as possible after purchase. In addition, they should be stored away from sunlight.

Vitamin B3 (Nicotinamide)

Studies have shown that vitamin B3 may be able to combat some of the antibiotic resistant staphylococcal infections.

Research has shown that high doses of this vitamin increased by up to 1,000 times the ability of the immune cells to kill staphylococcal bacteria.

These findings were published in the *Journal of Clinical Investigation* on August 27 by researchers from the Linus Pauling Institute at Oregon State University, UCLA and other institutions.

Vitamin B3 stimulates the innate immune system to provide a much more powerful response. In the case of vitamin B3, clinical doses of this increased the numbers and effectiveness of neutrophils. These white blood cells kill and eat harmful bacteria.

NEUTROPHIL

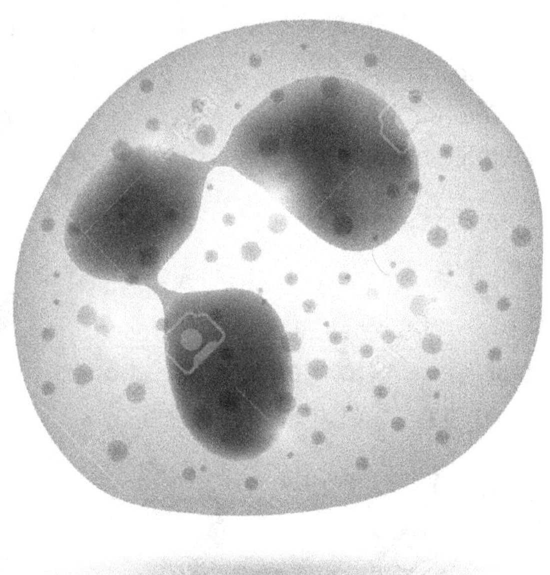

Further studies showed that clinical doses of vitamin B3 appeared to wipe out the staph infection in only a few hours.

It is not recommended that megadoses of this vitamin are taken routinely, without medical supervision, since high doses of vitamin B3 can damage the liver.

Given the potential negative side effects of mega doses of vitamin B3, a healthy balanced diet containing whole grains, mushrooms, peanuts, avocados and green peas should be the aim. This will provide the recommended daily allowance for vitamin B3 of:

- 14mg for women
- 16mg for men.

Higher doses are available via prescription but are normally given to help lower cholesterol levels rather than to treat staph infections.

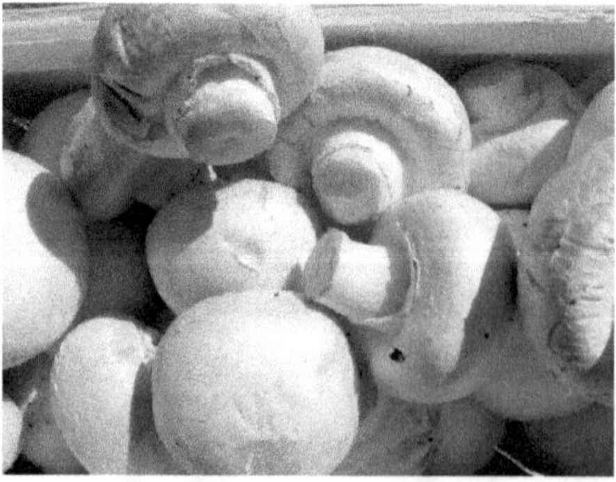

Mushrooms contain vitamin B3 and can help fight staphylococcus infections.

Nutritional yeast is a great source of B vitamins including vitamin B3.

Mushrooms

It is perhaps fitting that we finished off the last section showing that mushrooms had the potential to kill off an enveloped bacterium[7]. Mushrooms are thought to be one of the richest sources of natural antibiotics. It is thought that they evolved this way as they had to protect themselves from the often damp and dirty environment that they grow in.

Many prescribed antibiotics are made from mushrooms. These include streptomycin and tetracycline. For example, Ganomycin, a powerful antibiotic is made from Reishi mushrooms. However, most mushrooms will have both antibacterial and antiviral properties although these will be of greater or lesser strength depending on the variety of mushroom.

---

[7] Enveloped bacterium include staphylococcus aureus, streptococcus pneumoniae, enterococcus faecalis

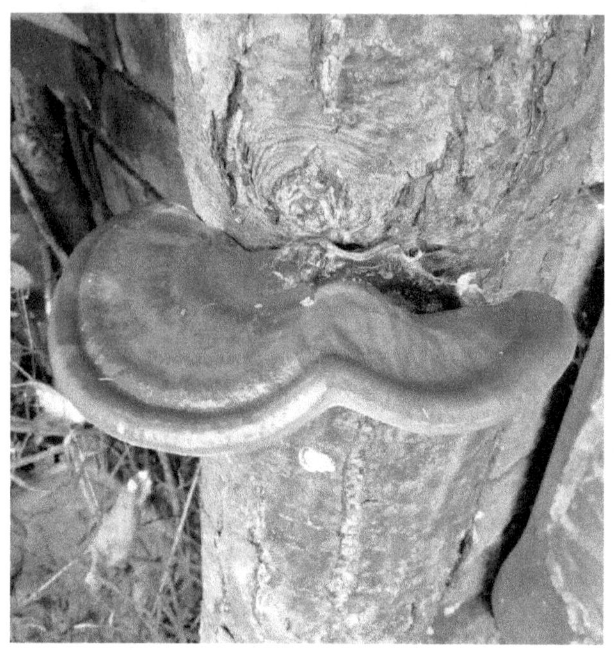

Ganomycin is made from Reishi mushrooms [8]

Ganomycin has also been found to be helpful in the treatment of metabolic resistance assisting in weight loss, insulin resistance, hypoglycaemia and hepatic steatosis.

Reishi mushroom is also capable of boosting your immune system and some forms of reishi are capable of altering inflammation pathways in white blood cells.

[8] https://www.gourmetmushrooms.co.uk/shop/plug-spawn/reishi-mushroom-plug-spawn/

Research in cancer patients[9] has shown that some of the molecules found in the mushroom can increase the activity of a white blood cell which is part of the innate immune system. These are called Natural Killer cells (NK's).

Natural killer cells fight cancer and infections in the body. Other studies have shown that reishi can increase the number of lymphocytes in those with colorectal cancer.[10]

Lymphocytes are white cells that are vital to our immune system defences. There are three main types:

- T cells
- B cells
- Natural killer cells

Lymphocytes recognise invaders, produce antibodies and destroy any cells which could cause damage to us.

Reishi potentially has cancer fighting properties. One study showed that of over 4,000 breast cancer survivors, 59% of them consumed reishi mushrooms.

---

[9] https://www.ncbi.nlm.nih.gov/pubmed/12916709
[10] https://www.ncbi.nlm.nih.gov/pubmed/16428086

Other studies[11] did not find this link between reishi and anti-cancer effects although they did find an improved response to chemotherapy in those eating reishi.

It is thought that reishi should be used as an adjunctive therapy alongside traditional cancer treatment.

The five best mushrooms with antiviral and antibacterial efficacy were found to be:

.

- Coliolus
- Reishi
- Shiitake
- Mitake
- Agarikon

Coliolus was found to be effective against both gram + and gram- bacteria. In S *aureus,* extracts from coliolus were found to elongate and cause malformation of their cells.   In Salmonella Enteritidis, colilolus was found to rupture the cells walls thus killing the bacterium.

---

[11] https://www.cancertherapyadvisor.com/fact-sheets/cancer-reishi-mushroom-fact-sheet/article/647081/2/

Shiitake mushrooms were tested against 29 bacterial and fungal pathogens. It was found that there was extensive antimicrobial activity against 85% of these pathogens.

The antiviral and antibacterial effects came from such substances like:

- Oxalic acid
- Lentinan
- Centinanycins A and B
- Eritadenine (antiviral)

Agarikon is a huge fungus which hangs off trees

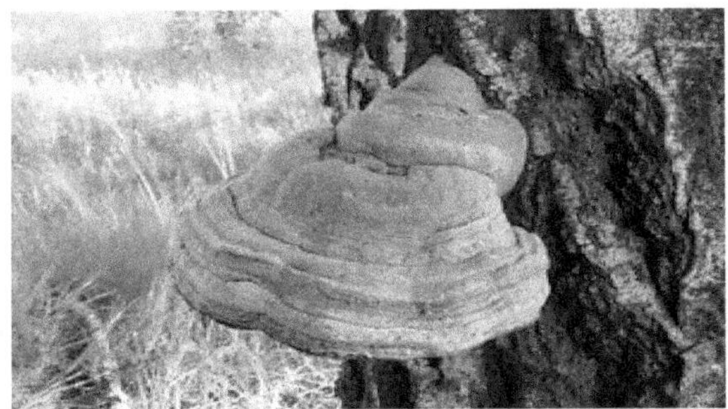

Studies show that Agarikon showed efficacy against tuberculosis and that it also reduced inflammation as well as many other bacterial and viral infections. It shows strong activity against cowpox, swine and bird flu and the virus that causes herpes. Mycologist, Paul Stamets, noted that agarikon's effectiveness was better, in some cases, than conventional therapies.[12]

There are many powdered forms of mushroom on the market which can be bought through health food shops or online and which can be made into a tea, soup or added to a vegetable terrine, as wished. Be guided by the instructions on the packet and, if any side effects do occur then reduce the amount you are using. However, studies of reishi mushroom, in particular, show very few side effects, even when it has been used for an extended time.

---

[12] : https://phys.org/news/2014-10-mycologist-agarikon-possibility-counter-antibiotic.html#jCp

The healing power of garlic

Garlic has long been recognised as having antibacterial and antiviral properties but its ability to deal with infective agents goes well beyond this. Garlic is a broad spectrum antibiotic and its efficacy extends to antifungal

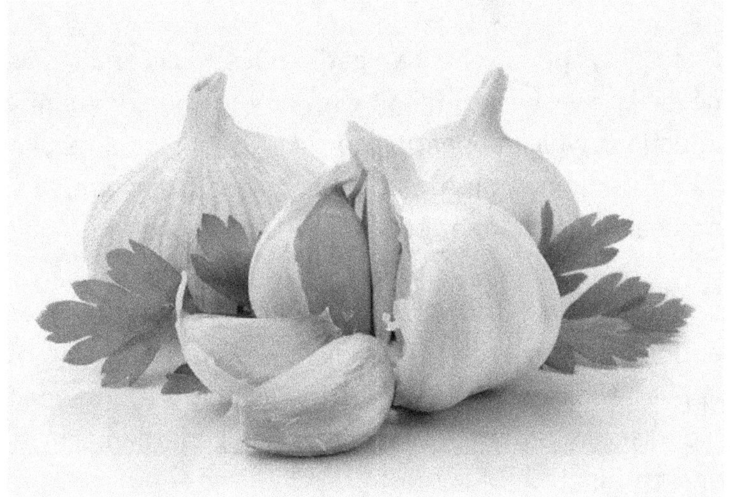

13

antiparasitic and antiprotozoan as well.

---

[13] http://humansarefree.com/2014/03/study-garlic-shrinks-tumors-up-to-74.html

Garlic is a bulb from the allium family and is well known for producing pungent breath when it has been eaten.

The active ingredient in garlic is allicin. It has to be eaten raw – not cooked – as heat will destroy or damage the enzymes thus rendering them ineffective against foreign invaders.

One of my friends eats two garlic cloves daily and I have never known him to fall ill with any of the community infections which appear to do their rounds on a regular basis. Garlic has the potential to lower blood pressure and has antioxidant effects, too.

Studies[14] have shown that garlic appears to have antibiotic activity whether it is taken internally or applied topically. Researchers found that the urine and blood serum of human subjects taking garlic had activity against fungi.

Many pharmaceutical antibiotics promote the development of resistant strains of bacteria. Garlic does not appear to produce these resistant strains of bacteria. Further, it may be effective against strains which have become resistant to pharmaceutical antibiotics.

---

[14] Caporaso et al 1983

Moore and Atkins (1977) tested garlic juice against a group of ten different bacteria and yeasts. They found that garlic was effective against all of them and they also found 'a complete absence of development of resistance.'

Garlic has also found to be effective against specific bacteria that are notorious for developing resistant strains such as staphylococcus, mycobacterium, salmonella and species of Proteus.

As antibiotics aren't effective against viruses, then they aren't effective against colds and flu. The viruses responsible for colds and influenzas are able to change shape so that they aren't fully recognised if they invade a body again. This explains why it is possible to suffer repeated colds and flu.

In contrast, most people who get the common childhood illnesses like measles, mumps and chicken pox rarely get them more than once since these viruses a retain more stable structure. And do not readily morph into something that the body has not recognised in the past. As such, if a stable virus tries to invade a second time, the body recognises it immediately. Antibody defences are available immediately to deal with it – and we are unlikely to have any symptoms.

Garlic has been found to work against influenza, herpes, cowpox, vesicular stomach virus, (cold sores) and cytomegalovirus (a common secondary infection found in those with AIDS).

In an animal study,[15] researchers fed a garlic extract to some mice. They then introduced the flu virus into the nasal passages of the mice. The control group did not receive any diet of garlic.

The mice fed the garlic were protected from the flu but the ones who didn't receive the garlic became sick.

The researchers hypothesised that the effects of garlic were partly due to its antiviral effects and partly due to stimulation of the immune system.

Garlic activates phagocytes which engulf invading pathogens. It helps stimulate B cells and T cells. This is all at the level of the cellular immune system.

Garlic contains a substance known as diallyl trisulphide. This activates natural killer cells and macrophages. It also increases B-cell activity which subsequently increases the antibodies which attach themselves to pathogens and mark them for destruction.

---

[15] Adetumbi and Lau 1983

Diallyl trisulphide treated macrophages were also found to be more active against cancer cells than macrophages not treated with diallyl-trisulphide. Not only was their number increased but their activity was too.[16] Studies with patients suffering from AIDS showed that two cloves a day given to ten patients for six weeks followed by four cloves of garlic for another six weeks revealed normal levels of natural killer cells when previously they had been low.

Opportunistic infections – infections which take advantage of a lowered immune system – such as sinusitis and pneumonia – improved. What is telling is that the patient with sinusitis[17] had not gained any relief from antibiotics.

Another study showed that a preparation of garlic powder given to elderly patients showed an increase in phagocytosis of the white blood cells ad also increased the number of lymphocytes. This is good news for those with pneumonia.

These are the main nutrients that the patient was supplemented with. Supplements were important because the effort of breathing makes eating very difficult and it would be well- nigh impossible to take

---

[17] Abdullah 1989

the amount of nutrients required to act therapeutically.

Eating tiny amounts, often with supplements, is what was required and accepted at the time.

Four days into the second course of antibiotics and intense course of supplements, my husband patient was up and pottering around and had regained his appetite. The change was quite remarkable.

There have been improvements in food intake, interest in surroundings, ability to talk in sentences without breathlessness and ability to self-care when such treatments are initiated if pneumonia strikes. However, such measures like keeping optimum levels of vitamin C and vitamin D all year round is a major preventative measure.

Pneumonia takes up to six months to fully recover from but the phrase 'fully recover from' will apply only if the underlying pneumonia is dealt with properly and swiftly. It is even better if it can be avoided altogether. Susceptible people must therefore take stock of their diet and the need to have therapeutic doses of beneficial supplements to hand should any infection start.

In my husband's case, once he was home and we could start supplements (hospitals never allow these) he was back to being busy within the week. He had remarked on returning home that he the consultant said it would take months to recover properly.   Well, we proved him wrong.

How did infection start?

In my husband's case, the general malaise and slight heaviness in breathing were the only initial signs. Certainly observations did not immediately show up anything for concern. Therefore, do not wait for an increase in temperature or the breathing rate to increase before you start taking therapeutic doses of supplements. By that time the infection will have taken hold properly.

It will not harm if therapeutic doses of vitamins and minerals are taken only to find out that they probably were not needed.

It is always better to be safe than sorry.

Carvacrol

The increase of resistant strains of bacteria and other infective agents have made it a necessity to find new classes of antibacterial compounds that inhibit the defensive mechanisms found in bacteria.

Oregano oil has been found to be one such compound. It contains a phenolic compound known as carvacrol. It has a broad spectrum of antimicrobial activity in addition to being:

- Anti-inflammatory
- Antioxidant
- Anti-tumour
- Antitussive
- Antispasmodic
- Anti-leishmanial (protects against a specific parasite)
- Hepatoprotective (protects against liver damage)

It is effective against gram positive and gram negative bacteria.

Studies included a Minimum inhibitory concentration (M IC) test which determined the lowest concentration of Carvacrol needed to inhibit visible (99%) bacterial growth after overnight incubation,

The mean value was obtained from three tests.

The carvacrol was analysed in different concentration against inhibition of:

- S aureus
- S epidermis
- St Pneumonia
- Klebsiella pneumonia

among others. The Streptococcus Pneumoniae bacterium is responsible for most pneumonias.

There are nearly 100 different strains of this type (known as serotypes) and they are to be found on a continuum from mild to severe. However, the severity of any serotype should also be considered in context. In an elderly malnourished patient even a mild serotype may produce a severe illness. You cannot afford to neglect the nutrients required for optimum immune system functioning.

Anti-microbial effects were seen and the growth of bacteria was found to be inhibited in different sites of infection including *St Pneumoniae* and Klebsiella pneumonia.

The mode of action of carvacrol appears to be its ability of disintegrate the outer membrane of bacterial cells of gram negative bacteria releasing lipopolysaccharides (LPS).

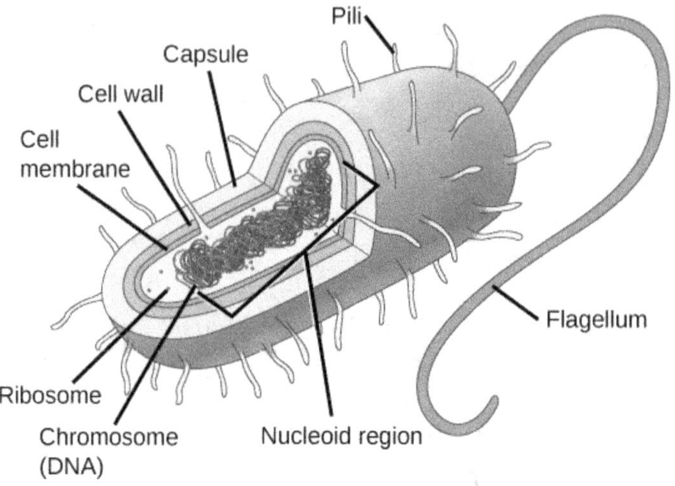

It also increases the permeability of the membrane around the cytoplasm to ATP.

Used as a spray for sore throats, it is reported that it relieved pain within 20 minutes. In addition, due to its analgesic effects, it alleviated muscle aches commonly found in flu.

The ability of carvacrol and other phenolic compounds to damage membrane and arrest growth in both grams positive and negative bacteria should not be underestimated.

Sprinkling a little dried oregano on top of a dish is unlikely to have any therapeutic effect. There are supplements Which can be bought online which come in a pearl sized form. They contain 25mg each and the recommended dosage can be found on the packet.

If you feel that a higher dosage would be beneficial then consult a nutritionist. Phenolic acids such as carvacrol can thin the blood   and while this is useful in infections which increase the risk of blood clotting, it needs discussing with a nutritionist who understands this property of phenolic acids.

Copper – deadly antiviral

Copper as an anti-infective agent has been recognised as such for over 2,000 years. Hippocrates recommended it to people to prevent infections of any sort.

Copper oxide and copper ions need only 6 hours to inactivate influenza A, virus particles. Copper destroys their genetic material by interacting with oxygen and preventing mutation. In addition, it inhibits attachment of the virus to the host cell so that infection cannot take hold.

It is capable of killing every known strain of virus including the Coronavirus. Indeed, Coronavirus was found to be permanently and rapidly deactivated when in contact with copper.

Using this concept, a device known as the Copper Zap was invented in the US. At the first sign of a cold, the Copper Zap can be inserted into the nostrils for a short time where it will rapidly kill viruses.

Other individuals make a gargle using copper supplements at the first sign of a sore throat.

However, it is judicious to maintain a diet which contains adequate amounts of copper, bearing in mind that high levels of zinc and vitamin C can also deplete copper over time.

Foods which contain good amounts of copper include:

- Liver
- Oysters
- Nuts and seeds
- Lobster
- Dark leafy greens
- Dark chocolate

The recommended dietary allowance is 900mcg daily. However, a word of caution is required here – a deficiency or excess of copper can have negative side effects so supplementation is not recommended unless under medical supervision. Further, if copper is not bound to a

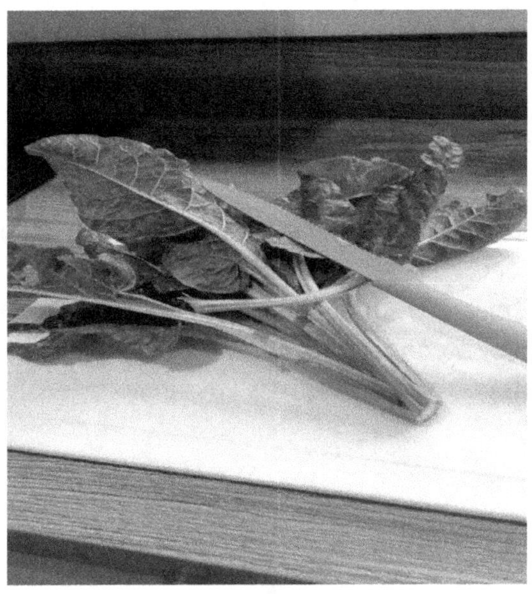

Dark green leafy vegetables contain good amounts of copper.

protein – which occurs in food as a matter of course – then it has toxic properties. For example, the copper found in supplements is generally a salt of copper – that is an unbound form. I cannot recommend supplements of copper unless you know for certain that they are in a non-labile form.

Copper from copper pipes used to convey drinking to households is also toxic and should be avoided. The best sources of copper are from food in a well-balanced diet.

Signs of a copper deficiency – other than frequent viral infections - include:

- abnormal skin and hair pigmentation
- iron deficient anaemia
- poorly functioning immune system resulting in bacterial infections
- poor memory and lack of creative thinking.
- Poor connective tissue formation. Copper is required for the cross links in collagen.

Selenium

While most people are acquainted with the positive benefits of vitamin C and D on infection, most people have not heard of selenium, never mind have an idea of which foods It can be found in.

Selenium is a trace mineral which means that you only require it in small amounts. Selenium helps make tiny proteins known as antioxidant enzymes. These help to prevent cell damage.

The health of the immune system is dependent on obtaining adequate amounts of selenium which lowers oxidative stress thus reducing inflammation and increasing immunity.

Studies have confirmed that enhanced blood levels of this trace mineral result in a better immune response. A deficiency has been shown in studies to slow the immune response. Benefits or those with TB, hepatitis C and influenza have been found.

Many viruses like the enveloped ones responsible for influenza and coronavirus, have the ability to mutate easily. However, mutations appear to occur only in those hosts who have a selenium deficiency. The mutations that occur resulted in increased virulence. Thus mutations and spread of virus appear to be related to selenium status in the host.

Selenium deficiency is rife due to selenium deficient soils that plants are grown in.

However, two brazil nuts will supply the day's allowance of selenium.

In addition, other foods which contain good amounts of selenium are:

- Chicken and turkey
- Beef and pork
- Fish and shellfish
- Mushrooms
- Beans
- Some fruit and vegetables
- Brewer's yeast

BUT anything grown in selenium deficient soil would not contain that level of selenium that we would expect. In addition, any animal grazing on selenium deficient land may also lack this nutrient in the amounts that we would expect in the meat.

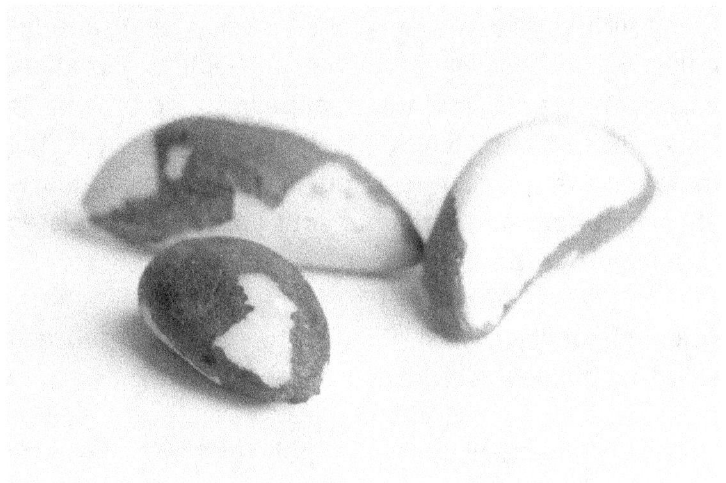

Brazil nuts are by far the best source of selenium

Vitamin E

While most people are aware that vitamin C and D are useful in preventing or reducing symptoms of infection, I never hear people say this of vitamin E. However, there are many studies showing that vitamin E may reduce the incidence of bacterial and viral infections.

One such study[18] looked at the benefits of increasing vitamin E in relation to pneumonia in elderly males. The participants were male smokers aged 50-69 and they were given 50mg/d of vitamin E for 5-8 years.

Out of 2,216 participants, the study showed that vitamin E supplementation reduced the incidence of pneumonia by 69%. Even a further group who smoked greater amounts of cigarettes had a significantly reduced incidence of pneumonia.

Mouse studies[19] have also found that extra vitamin E can protect against a common type of   bacterial pneumonia. It appeared that extra vitamin E helped regulate the mice's immune system. This study which was initially published online in the Journal of Immunology is useful when investigating the effects of vitamin E on bacterial pneumonia in humans.

The regulation of the immune system is vital in preventing the damage that may occur in elderly individuals. Neutrophils – kamikaze white cells which make a one way trip to destroy infection – can destroy lung tissue if they are not regulated properly.

---

[18]
https://pubmed.ncbi.nlm.nih.gov/27757026/#:~:text=Background%3A%20Vitamin%20E%20has%20influenced,supplementation%20on%20pneumonia%20in%20humans.
[19] https://www.infectioncontroltoday.com/view/can-extra-vitamin-e-protect-against-common-type-pneumonia

Unfortunately, the ageing process reduces this regulatory process but, in the lungs of ageing mice, dietary vitamin E regulated the entry of neutrophils into murine lungs thus reducing inflammation which can destroy lung tissue.

The mice were studied before and after infection with the pneumonia causing bacteria. The mice had been fed differing amounts of vitamin E (alpha-tocopherol) over a 4 -week period. The control group were fed the recommended amounts while the experimental group were fed the equivalent of what would be ten times higher in humans.

It was found that the mice fed the diet higher in vitamin E were far more resistant to bacterial pneumonia than those fed the normal amounts normally recommended. It was found that the mice fed the extra vitamin E had one thousandth   fewer bacteria in their lungs. In addition, they had half as many neutrophils.

The outcome of this was that the reduction in bacteria and neutrophils had a knock on effect on the health of lung tissue. Infection seemed to be dealt with as well as a younger mouse would deal with it.

Indeed, growing numbers of research point towards Vitamin E as the nutrient that can ameliorate the loss of the immune response caused by ageing.

Studies like these are important because as antibiotic resistance grows we are running out of antibiotics that can treat this condition. As nearly one million Americans will get pneumonia yearly with 400,000 hospitalised and 50,000 dying, then the burden on health systems and the impact on patients is high. Recovery from pneumonia is slow, even more so in the elderly.

The Recommended Daily Allowance for vitamin E is 400 IU's daily but clearly higher doses are required at times of bacterial infection.

Good sources of vitamin E are:

- Wheat germ
- Nuts
- Dark green leafy vegetables
- Sunflower seeds
- Beet greens
- Avocado's
- Whole wheat products
- Many vegetable oils

Vitamin E is a fat soluble vitamin and needs to be taken with a little fat to be absorbed.

Useful instruments to help diagnosis

GP's always have useful gadgets which they wrap around your arm or place on the end of your finger. If you are fairly confident and able to read figures when using gadgets, then there are a couple that you may find useful to buy. They are relatively inexpensive and worth their weight in gold.

The most useful gadget that I have found is the **oximeter.** If you have had chest infections before you will have experienced a small machine placed on the end of your finger. It measures the amount of oxygen in the blood and sometimes also checks your pulse rate.

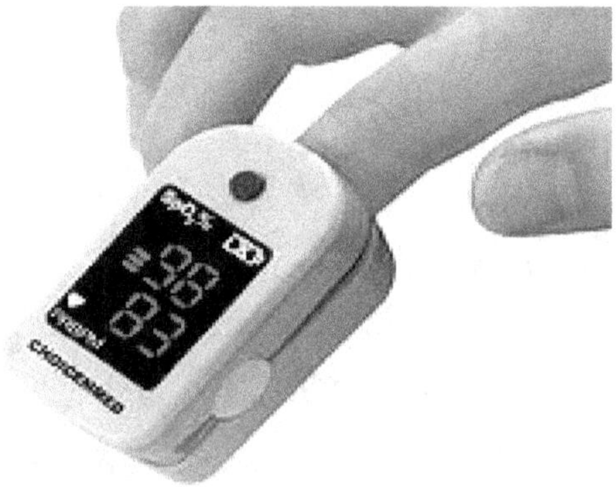

The optimum amount of oxygen in the blood is 99% and we do not like it to go below 90% as that can be damaging to brains and organs.

People with respiratory disease, like asthma may find theirs slightly lower than 99% (which is why they take inhalers to give maximum oxygen flow).

Oximeters are useful because they cannot only track your current SATS but also show if it is dropping.

The pulse rate is a useful tool. High heart rate is known as tachycardia and this   mainly occurs during infection or allergy. So, if your pulse rate is normally 70 and then during times of unwellness, it rises to 100 or above, then this is considered to be tachycardia and needs to be addressed as a matter of urgency.

 Never under-estimate the benefits of owning   a **thermometer.** The ones that can be used by briefly inserting in the outer ear or pointed at the forehead, are the easiest and quickest to use. However, they also tend to be the most expensive.

Normal temperature is 37C but a couple of degrees either way is not a matter of concern. Temperature rises briefly after taking in food, wearing too much clothing and exercising. The time of the day can also affect this. Thermometers often come with a traffic light guide which is a helpful aid in ascertaining whether anything is untoward.

A fever normally starts at 38C and this indicates that your body is fighting infection.

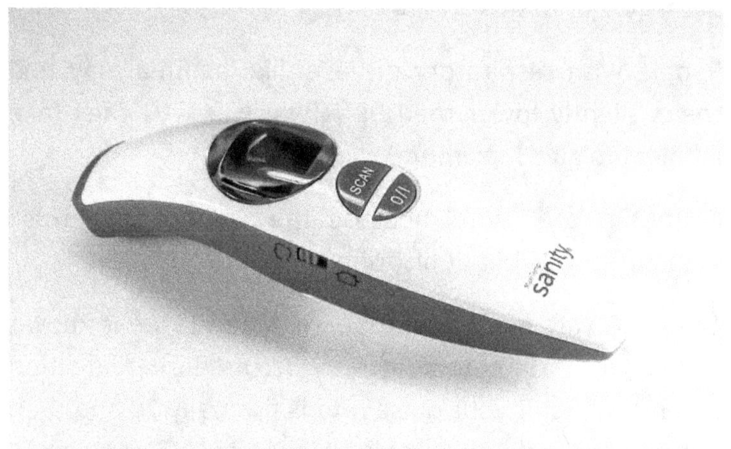

The reading of the 'gun' thermometer is almost instantaneous and more accurate than the thermometers that you place under your tongue or armpit. True they are more expensive, but poorly patients appreciate not being attached to gadgets longer than is absolutely necessary.

When a person is unwell, it is useful in the early stages to undertake regular temperature and oxygen/pulse rate checks so you can see if the infection is progressing or receding. It helps to record this. It is very easy to forget things when there are numerous checks to be undertaken, medication to be dispensed. Pneumonia can disrupt memory so do not rely on the patient to be able to recall what checks and medications have been completed.

A **sphygmometer** is simply another name for a blood pressure machine. The cuff wraps neatly around your upper arm and records the upper (systolic) and lower (diastolic) number. The normal reading is 120/80.

Some medics believe that blood pressure will rise with age. It generally does but it is not 'normal' in that respect. It simply indicates that you are ageing or have arterial plaque or some such other thing going on which could be addressed so that further ill health does not occur.

Some people have naturally lower blood pressure. If they do they normally have longer lives - in terms of lack of cardiovascular events - because their heart does not have to work as hard to pump blood around the body. Therefore, it does not wear out quickly.

It does help to know what is 'normal' for you before you can begin to interpret what is going on.

In bacterial pneumonia, a condition called sepsis may arise.

Sepsis occurs when toxins are produced in certain bacteria. These toxins instruct cells in the body to release cytokines which cause inflammation.

Cytokines are useful because they help the immune system to fight infection but they can go overboard and get out of control (often because there is a vitamin D deficiency which modulates the immune system).

Cytokines [20]can cause blood vessels to dilate and cause a decrease in blood pressure. Often this can be quite dramatic. Such an occurrence may mean that there is not enough oxygen for the brain and organs of the body. This is serious.

So, it is helpful to know what your normal blood pressure, oxygen SATS and pulse rate are before you can begin to understand what is going on.

It is also helpful to have these figures to hand and records of any changes to give to any health or emergency services should you need to ring them.

---

[20] It is the cytokine storm that is responsible for most deaths in bacterial pneumonia. The inflammatory responses go overboard and the lungs are filled up with cells of the immune system impairing the ability of the exchange of gases,

Tests that may be ordered

I have covered some of the tests that may be ordered in previous chapters and some of the common ones that still haven't will be looked at below.

Bronchoscopy

This involves a direct examination of the bronchi.

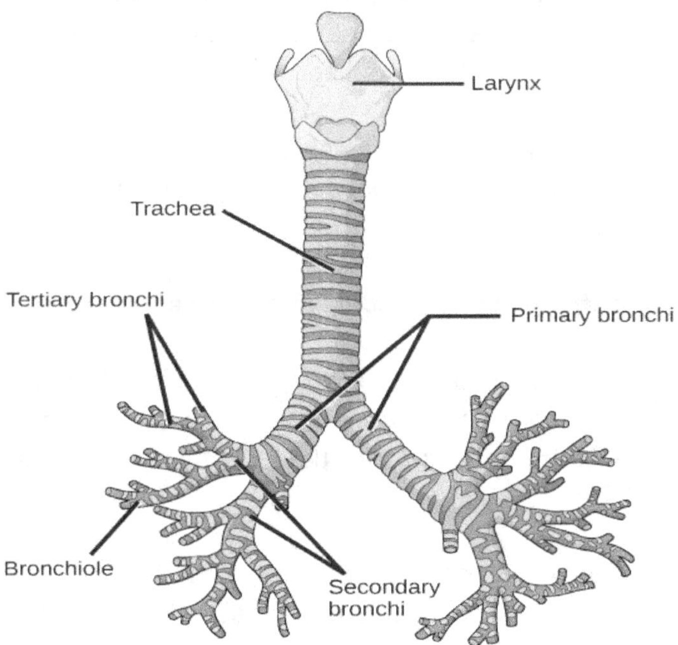

A bronchoscope is used. This is a flexible tube and it is useful in the diagnosis of lung conditions such as what blockages or narrowing there may be,

Bronchoscopes are also able take sample of fluid or tissue for further analysis.

Pleural fluid culture

There is a space between the chest wall and lungs known as the pleural space. Fluid is obtained from this area via a long needle attached to a syringe into which the fluid is pulled.

This has uses in establishing what bacterium is causing the infection. So that appropriate treatment can be started.

Other ways of avoiding pneumonia

Pneumonia often follows influenza which is why the flu jab is recommended. Influenza is a nasty infection and impairs the effectiveness of immune system.

 However, there are downsides to the flu vaccine in that respiratory infections that follow it tend to be more severe. There is good research to support this. Since pneumonia may follow on the back of any respiratory virus or weakened state, then having the flu vaccine does not necessarily mean that your chances of pneumonia are reduced. Any other normally mild respiratory virus may take on a more severe form post flu vaccination. This alone could damage the immune system's defences and allow pneumonia to take hold.

This phenomenon is known as Respiratory Virus Interference[21] (RVI)

The severity of Respiratory Virus Interference may differ depending on the viruses they subsequently encounter.

Another problem with the flu vaccine is that it has a low efficacy rate. Many people who have the vaccine will either not make any antibodies or not enough of them to create effective immunity. This is especially true of the older population. Generally, as we age, the immune system does not work as efficiently as a young healthy adult's. Whether this would also affect RVI is not entirely clear.

So, some questions you need to ask before your flu vaccination are:

- Is this vaccine a good match for this year's flu?
- What can I do to strengthen my immune system naturally?

---

[21] https://pubmed.ncbi.nlm.nih.gov/31607599/

- Do I need a pneumonia jab, first?

The pneumococcal vaccine protects against one of the more common forms of bacterial pneumonia but as we have seen there are many types of infection causing it. So yes, this vaccine would be useful but will not protect you from all forms of pneumonia.

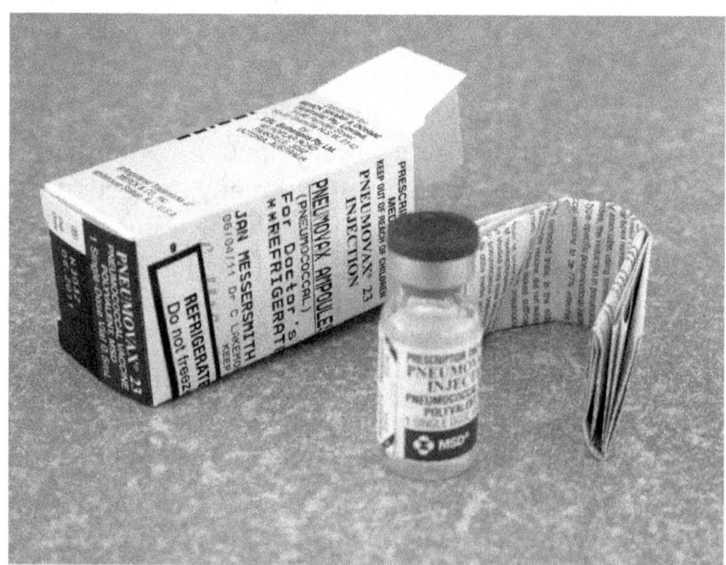

Normally pre-school children and those over 65 will be offered this shot and it can be topped up in the elderly every 5 years or so.

This shot can also be given to those outside this age group who have underlying health disorders which predispose them to infection like pneumonia.

If measures are taken to avoid pneumonia then associated conditions like respiratory failure, acute respiratory distress syndrome, lung abscesses and sepsis can be avoided.

Before we finish this book, it would be useful to understand what these mean for the patient.

Respiratory failure would indicate the need for a ventilator or breathing machine.

The symptoms of acute respiratory failure are:

In cases of high carbon dioxide levels

- Confusion and rapid breathing

Patients with low oxygen levels may experience

- Bluish tone to fingernails, skin and lips
- Being unable to breathe

Low oxygen levels and an acute failure of the lungs will result in:

- Anxiety
- Being sleepy
- Tachycardia
- Rapid shallow breathing
- Irregular heartbeats
- Loss of consciousness
- sweating

Lung abscesses – these are areas of pus which would need to be drained through surgical means.

Symptoms of lung abscess include:

- Chest pain especially when you breathe in
- Loss of appetite
- Night sweats
- Fever
- Fatigue
- Weight loss
- Sputum – this is a mixture of mucus and saliva containing pus which is often streaked with pus.

Acute respiratory distress syndrome (ARDS) – a more severe form of respiratory failure which comes on very rapidly

The symptoms of ARDS are:

- Fast breathing or taking lots of shallow, rapid breaths (normal breathing is between 7-9 breaths every half minute
- Fast heart rate (over 100 beats per minute)
- Shortness of breath
- A productive cough
- Blue tone to the skin or lips. This is not so easily discerned in those with darker skin. Look at the fingernails which will take on a blue tone.
- Crackling sound in the lungs
- Fever (over 38C)
- fatigue

Sepsis - the infection enters the blood stream and may lead to organ failure.

The symptoms of sepsis in the elderly include:

- Blotchy and/or discoloured skin
- Very low body temperature
- Fever and chills

- Fast heartbeat (tachycardia)
- Fatigue or weakness
- Diarrhoea
- Nausea and vomiting
- Lack of urination
- Slurred speech
- confusion

The after effects of pneumonia

Pneumonia can take a long time to recover from even after all the antibiotics, steroids and oxygen assistance is but a distant memory.

Previously fit and healthy people can be floored by pneumonia and this even more so in the elderly who take longer to recover.

Providing that there is no lasting damage such as lung scarring or a discovery of a malignancy, then complete recovery can occur but you need to be patient.

Even the act of washing yourself can leave you fatigued so you need to understand this. When you are feeling tired, then you need to stop and rest. Early to bed and late to rise is what is required interspersed with an afternoon doze.

Sleeping may not be easy especially if you have pain or fluid on the lungs. The latter makes it difficult to take proper deep breaths so that breathing is satisfying and complete.

Some people are able to sleep propped up on many pillows but this can be beyond some patients. They may have to sit upright packed into a favourite chair leaning forward onto a strategically placed pillow on a table.

You will note the milestones reached as the condition improves. The patient will go from sleeping upright to being propped up onto 5 pillows and then four and so on.

What a glorious day it is when you can move down to your usual number of pillows and be able to sleep on your side.

The cough that is so raucous and persistent in the morning will gradually soften and eventually disappear but it doesn't happen overnight.

The act of eating and drinking can leave a patient exhausted. Small amounts of nutritionally dense food and sips of water need to be offered on a regular basis and expect weight loss. I have nursed many patients who have had pneumonia and weight loss is the norm.

During the waking hours, - and in order to avoid the loss of muscle mass - a trip of twenty steps or so on an hourly basis will help prevent this loss. Small amounts of exercise will help to prevent blood clots as well as aid the circulation of lymph. The lymphatic system relies entirely on movement for its circulation. It does not have a pump like the heart does.

Bending toes down and up and flexing wrists in a similar fashion, while you are lying in bed, will help recovery. However, it has not to be done at all costs if you are tired.

For many days the route between chair and bed may be the only one you take. That is fine. Others need to do the shopping, make the beds and undertake the hoovering. One day, the patient will want to undertake some small task and that is a small sign that the lungs are healing well.

Expect breathlessness for some time. Even when all the patient's observations are all within normal limits and the SATS at 99% it is quite normal to exhibit some breathlessness. That will go in time.

The room should be kept warm but not stuffy. The patient needs a table nearby with all the things that they may require within reach.

Often patients feel guilty about the amount of time that others spend caring for them and do not like to bother the carer when they need something.

Meals should be small, nutritionally dense and tempting. Some of the protein powders that body builders use can provide lots of protein in a small serving but it is also necessary to provide fats and carbohydrates too.

Fats and oils aid the absorption of vitamin D and provide vitamin A - the latter of which is necessary for the health of the respiratory tract.

Yogurt and kefir may go down well and are excellent at helping replace gut bacteria lost when antibiotics were prescribed. Small chunks of banana provide fibre which help feed good gut bacteria.

Vegetables which have been left on a lovingly prepared plate may be acceptable if they are whizzed up into a soup. A little stock or milk added at the time adds to the nutritional status.

Home-made jelly has sound nutritional status containing the protein gelatine. Home-made is better because you can keep the sugar content low and use fresh juices. It slips down easily as does ice-cream.

People who normally enjoy cooking will be adept at adapting recipes for the occasion. For others the complete meal sachets may be useful. They do contain many added nutrients but probably not in the quantities need at times of recovering from a pneumonia.

Heart failure

Following a bout of pneumonia when recovery appears to be well on the way, quite marked oedema can occur. Sometimes this can be in one leg or both and in many cases it is first noticed when socks and shoes simply do not fit anymore.

Heart failure is simply the failure of the heart to be able to cope with the demands of the body at the time. Thus walking around shopping may be doable but walking uphill may be not.

Abdominal distension occurs due to oedema. Sometimes this may occur due to steroid medication. As a result, when this medication is stopped then some of the distension may go. However, the steroidal induced form does not readily revert to its previous shape although the abdominal protrusion may become less evident.

Sometimes though, nasty infections like pneumonia can result in heart failure. Heart failure can occur when the heart is unable to pump blood around the body properly. The heart has become stiff or weak.

Symptoms of heart failure are many. They include a persistent cough which is worse at night, wheezing, dizziness, confusion, bloated stomach, loss of appetite, weight gain (due to excess fluid) weight loss due to the effort it takes to eat, easy fatigue, a fast heart rate and palpitations.

Heart failure is silent for a long time. The tendency to fatigue, forgetfulness and weight gain can so easily be put down to so many things. If you don't feel like eating then of course you will lose weight but the loss of appetite is rarely, initially, put down to something like heart failure.

The symptoms can be treated but heart failure is not considered to be reversible. The prognosis used to be poor with deaths occurring within 2-5 years. Better knowledge and treatments have prolonged this four fold in some patients and, of course, we now realise that heart failure is not necessarily a permanent feature since it very much depends on the activity and whether this matches the heart's resources.

The condition, once diagnosed with blood tests, an ECG and echocardiogram is generally treated with ACE inhibitors or ARB's; maybe both.

Angiotensin -2 receptor blockers (also known as ARB's)

These medications tend to end in 'sarten' such as Irbesartan which is one that is commonly prescribed. ARB's are useful in that they help prevent damage to the kidneys due to diabetes.

Like many other medications for high blood pressure they lower blood pressure by widening blood vessels.

Their action blocks angiotensin, a substance which narrows blood vessels.

However, the side effects of ARB's carry a long list. These include:

sexual dysfunction

chest pain

musculoskeletal pain

indigestion

liver problems

increased heartbeat

hypersensitivity

vasculitis

muscle cramps

altered taste

tinnitus

Natural ARB's are plentiful and include:

potassium – you can see that if you take diuretics that a natural ARB may be in short supply

Taurine

Fibre

Celery

Co-enzyme Q10

Vitamin B6 (Pyroxidone)

Vitamin C

Garlic

Resveratrol

Omega 3 fatty acids

Pyrioxidine is one of the B complex vitamins.

Good sources of this vitamin are:

Pork

Poultry

Oats

Wheat germ

Peanuts

Soya beans

Bananas

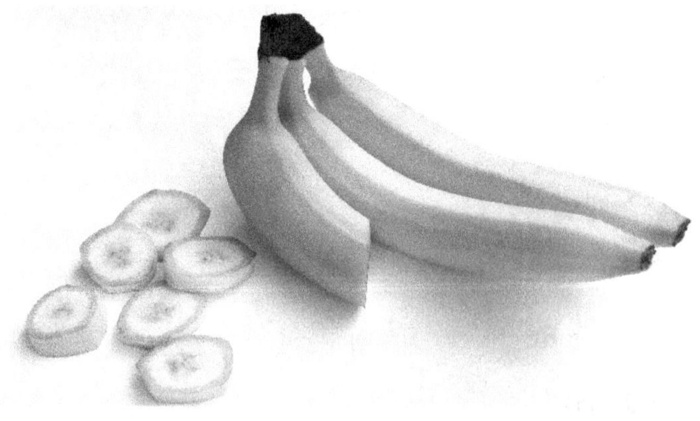

Bananas are a great source of Pyrioxidine, potassium and fibre and are able to contribute to the maintenance of normal blood pressure.

ACE inhibitors nearly always figure in treatment for hypertension and heart failure so the part on this type of medication is a little longer and more involved. There is some chemistry involved and some people will like this challenge and others not. If you are one of the latter, just pass it by and go onto the foods which can replace ACE inhibitors. It is not necessary for you to know how something works for it to work.

Angiotensin Converting Enzymes (ACE) (this part is taken from the book The Metabolic Syndrome Diet by Lynne D M Noble)

There are many different metabolic pathways responsible for blood pressure regulation by means of Angiotensin Converting Enzymes (ACE). They are related to the following systems

Renin-angiotensin (RAS) also known as the renin-angiotensin-aldosterone system

Renin-chymase (RCS)

Kinin-nitric oxide (KNOS)

Neutral endopeptide (NEPS)

The one we have already looked at in some detail is the RAS system.

There are many food-originating ACE inhibitors which include antihypertensive peptides.

Ace inhibitors derived from food proteins are the best known group of bioactive peptides

Dairy foods are excellent ACE Inhibitors.

They treat **primary hypertension** very well indeed.

Primary hypertension occurs due to life style factors like obesity and lack of exercise.

If you are not obese and take regular exercise, then this chapter may not have as much relevance for you. However, if you are obese and fell running does not appeal to you, then this chapter may be relevant to you.

Secondary hypertension occurs due other medical conditions like kidney disease.

Antihypertensive peptides differ slightly at each end.

At one end is attached an amine group and this is called the N-terminal.

The amino acid residue on the other end has a carboxylic acid group attached to it and this is referred to as the C-terminal

Thus for simplicity

N------ | peptide | ——————— **C**

There are specific amino acids residues which are typical for the N or C end of a peptide

The hydrophobic amino acids are characteristic of the N- end of a peptide and are specifically:

Glycine

Isoleucine

Leucine

valine

At the C end they are normally amino acids that are cyclic or have aromatic rings.

They comprise:

proline

tyrosine

tryptophan

We can make good use of this knowledge for it now means that foods containing the above amino acids inhibit ACE thus preventing a rise in blood pressure.

It might be better to tabulate the different amino acids and look at good sources in food.

Table showing N terminal amino acids and their food sources

Amino acid residue	Food sources
Isoleucine	Beef chicken pork fish dairy beans lentil legumes whole grains seeds cocoa dark chocolate

Leucine	Chicken beef pork fish tofu canned beans milk cheese squash seeds and eggs
valine	beef chicken pork fish tofu yogurt beans podded peas seeds nuts and whole grains
glycine	any gelatinous compounds like gelatine, bone broth, organ meats meat with the skin or crackling left on

Table showing C terminal amino acids and their food sources

Amino acid residue	Food sources
Proline	Gelatin, chicken skin

	pork crackling proline milk soy protein
Tyrosine	Beef pork fish chicken tofu milk cheese beans seeds nuts and whole grains bananas
Tryptophan	Nuts seeds tofu cheese red meat chicken turkey fish oats beans lentil and eggs bananas

You will see that some of these foods are ones we have been told to avoid because they are bad for us such as pork crackling. I do not agree that pork crackling is bad for you in moderation.

For further foods that contain these amino acids. Nutrition data website can provide information.

These foods all contain ACE inhibitors and should be eaten on a daily basis for those with primary hypertension.

For chocolate lovers who are feeling left out, chocolate also contains the amino acid phenylalanine. This has an association with tyrosine – one of our C-terminal amino acid residues.

Phenylalanine is involved in making dopamine which is a brain chemical than can regulate mood.

It helps to stimulate the metabolism firing up the processes that give life

You will note that the tables do not include simple carbohydrates purely because simple carbohydrates do not contain the amino acids that we require to inhibit ACE that narrows blood vessels.

At the end of this long passage on foods that can add to, or replace heart failure medications, we have learned some chemistry.

This stands us in good stead in understanding some of the many complex processes that underlie the mechanisms involving high blood pressure.

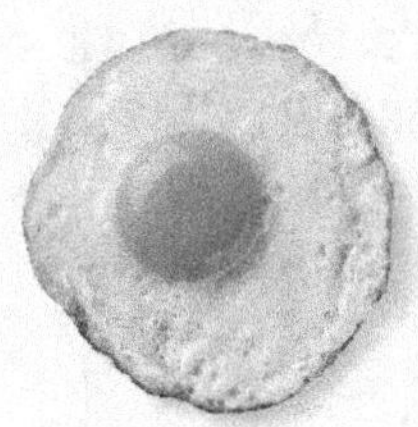

Eggs are a good source of N terminal amino acids

There are nutrients that have a vital part to play in reducing the impact and progression of heart failure.

We have met some of them briefly but it is now time to revisit them to look at how they have a role to play in the treatment of heart failure.

Taurine

Taurine has a major role to play in cardiovascular disease.   This amino acid is a physiological antagonist of HOCl which is a reactive form of oxygen.   HOCl is known to activate platelets and induce thrombosis.

Thrombotic complications are known to occur in 11-44% of those with congestive heart failure.

A study [22] of 14 patients found a therapeutic effect of taurine in congestive heart failure. These patients were divided into two groups – one of which had taurine supplementation and the other group took a placebo.

The taurine group did not have any patients that worsened over a 4-week period. However, 4 in the placebo group did.

As oily fish is a great source of taurine then those with heart failure may like to include it in their diets more.

---

[22] https://onlinelibrary.wiley.com/doi/pdf/10.1002/clc.4960080507

6g – in divided doses - was given in the above study.

Normally, the daily intake is between 500mg – 2000mg. It is a safe amino acid with low toxicity.

Mackerel contains about 78mg of taurine per 100g.

It would be hard to have a high intake of 6g through food alone but taurine supplements are available online or in health food shops and, given their benefits, cheap.

Here is a table of selected foods containing taurine[23]

---

[23] https://suppversity.blogspot.com/2010/08/taurine-from-foods-can-i-be-taurine.html

Food	Amount	Taurine (mg)
Cheese	3 ounces	1000
Cheese,cottage	1 cup	1700
Milk,whole	1 cup	400
Yogurt	1 cup	400
Wild game	3 ounces	600
Pork	3 ounces	540
Granola	1 cup	650
Oatmeal flakes	1 cup	500
Chocolate	1 cup	400
Meat (luncheon)	1 cup	390
Wheat germ,toasted	1/4 cup	350
Egg	1 (medium size)	350
Turkey	3 ounces	240
Duck	3 ounces	240
Chicken	3 ounces	185
Sausage	3 ounces	185
Avocado	1/2 (medium)	75

Having gained knowledge about the vital role taurine has in slowing down heart failure, we can now turn our attention to an enzyme that we have already met – that of coenzyme Q10 (hereinafter referred to as Q10).

Research has shown that   long term therapy with Q10 improves heart failure symptoms.

The study divided participants into two groups. One group received 100mg of Q10 three times daily and the second group, a placebo.

Participants were followed for two years.

The results showed that there was a significant improvement in functional parameters, ejection fraction, stroke volume and cardiac output in those who had the Q10.

The more a person was deficient in Q10 the greater the severity of heart failure symptoms. This statement has application to those who are on statins.

If statins are prescribed, then it is judicious to supplement with Q10.

The role of copper in cardiovascular disease

Studies have shown that improvements in the symptoms of heart failure have occurred when copper supplementation has been taken.

The Western diet is often deficient in copper and this may increase due to ageing for a number of reasons.

As people age their appetites often diminish, some of the foods that contain copper – red meat, for example - may not be easy to chew and, of course, the absorption of nutrients as we age, is not as efficient as it once was.

A diet deficient in copper will elevate blood pressure, cholesterol, homocysteine and uric acid. Further, it impairs glucose intolerance, promotes thrombosis and oxidative damage.

Copper supplementation is able to reverse the pleural effusion, heart failure and cardiac enlargement that occurs with a copper deficiency.

In addition to a lack of foods containing copper in the diet, a copper deficiency can also occur if there is too much zinc in the diet so any supplementation of copper should ideally take place well away from any zinc supplementation – a four hours' gap would be suitable.

I am not in favour of copper supplementation though. The copper contained in supplements is often a salt of copper. If copper is not attached to a protein source, then it may have detrimental effects on delicate brain tissue.

The best sources of copper are shellfish but these are not generally the mainstay of most people's diets. Organ meats are also rich in copper as are nuts, seeds, dark chocolate and wheat bran.

Beans are also a useful source of copper. About 100g of kidney beans contains 12% of your daily requirements.

Most people use beans in savoury dishes but mashed up with ingredients in a fruit cake, for example add to the richness of the flavour and produce a moister cake in addition to providing nutrients that you would not normally find there.

We have now not only come to the end of this chapter on nutrients that specifically can improve the symptoms of those with heart failure, but we have come to the end of this book.

As you may have come to realise, recovery from pneumonia is not a straightforward affair. Even after the patient has returned home from hospital, it is not unusual to find that there can be a long lasting impact on some vulnerable people that antibiotics simply cannot address.   This would include heart failure.

The post pneumonia x-ray that takes place approximately 6 weeks after infection may indicate that the infection has gone but that does not mean that the damage originally induced by the infection is over.

The British Lung Foundation has given an idea of what to expect if everything run smoothly.

1 week	your fever should be gone
4 weeks	your chest will feel better and you'll produce less mucus
6 weeks	you'll cough less and find it easier to breathe
3 months	most of your symptoms should be gone, though you may still feel tired
6 months	you should feel back to normal

Pneumonia can floor most people – even the fittest of people so although most people want to get back to normal as quickly as possible, you should impress upon others, who may demand your time, that you will be taking care of yourself as a priority.

During that time take walks when you are able to build up your lung function but equally, take extra rest and make sure your food is light but nutritious.

If you find that your symptoms are not going or new symptoms such as weight gain, weight loss or oedema are added then you must return to your GP. As this would indicate some post pneumonia problems that may need some extra care.

However, I am hopeful that adequate and bespoke nutrition will address any issues in a timely fashion with the exception of those patients who, during investigations, have been found to have other underlying conditions, which would impact on recovery and would need to be treated.

Three Years Later

In the last three years, those who I know have had regular bouts of pneumonia have been asked to follow the nutritional guidance in this book and, to date, none, who did follow the guidance, have suffered a recurrence of pneumonia. Indeed, many report feeling more invigorated than they ever did before their first bout.

Most report not having had any form of respiratory illness since following the measures contained in this book

Those diagnosed with heart failure have found it has not advanced. They have introduced extra taurine into their diet either through increasing oily fish or via supplementation. We forget – or have never been taught - the therapeutic effects of amino acids; they are a therapeutic treatment in themselves. Everything is there, we just need to learn and apply it. It used to be 'Granny's wisdom' but was taken away from us when more profitable remedies hit the supermarket shelves.

Addendum

All my books contain details of some of the charities or organisations that have made a profound and positive impact in their communities and beyond.

In some cases, they receive a percentage of the royalties generated from the sale of my books. In other cases, the information about the work that they undertake is disseminated more widely.

I have great pleasure in introducing you to Helping Hands Group Support and the sterling work that it does in supporting those who are struggling with life.

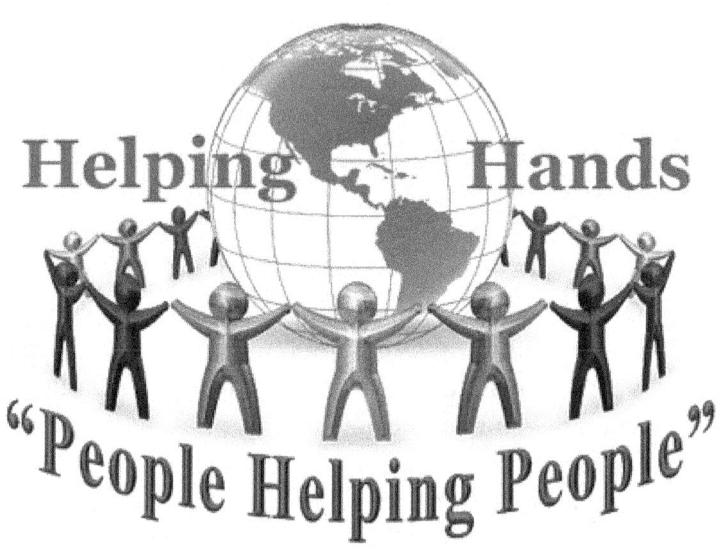

This group was the brainchild of Kerry. Kerry set up
Helping Hands Group Support after being inundated by
many on how to deal with 'injustices' caused by
government departments.

The group currently has 5000 supporters with more
being added daily. In addition, to their website, they
also have groups on Facebook, Telegram, Parler and
Twitter.

This group provides free template letters, free support,
free services and guidance to everyone to anyone who
requires it.

Kerry has recently brought on board Steve who is a fully
qualified senior electronics engineer who has over forty

years' experience in all and anything to do with electronics engineering and his expertise includes EMF, Communications etc

Steve is also well versed in   Human Rights and Laws and is also a qualified NEBOSH Health and Safety so this group can offer a wide range of support.

For more information on this please follow this link

https://www.facebook.com/Helpinghandsgroupsupport)

Other books by this author include:

- The EDS and Hypermobility Syndrome Diet
- Alleviating Symptoms of EDS
- Gastroparesis
- The EDS recipe book
- The Lipoedema Diet
- The Lymphoedema Diet: reverse and repair lymphatic damage
- The Anti Virus Diet
- The Asthma Diet
- The Reluctant Bowel
- The MND Diet
- Why we live longer with higher cholesterol levels

- A dietary connection for MACS, POTS and EDS
- Identity: a self-exploration workbook *
- Journey Through Pneumonia
- https://www.amazon.co.uk/dp/B07TBHMV6N

*This book can be used alone or in small group work and is an excellent resource for those who are 'people helpers.'

Among many others

They are available on Amazon

Lynne has written a semi-autobiographical trilogy.

While this trilogy is available on kindle and paperback on Amazon, it may be cheaper to buy from the link below.

They may be obtained off the publisher's website, in paperback form, where they are more reasonably priced.

https://www.shieldcrest.co.uk/?s=lynne+d+m+noble++

For the full range of books by this author, visit the author website on

https://www.amazon.co.uk/-/e/B07BPQZ5CD

https://www.amazon.com/-/e/B07BPQZ5CD

The Patient

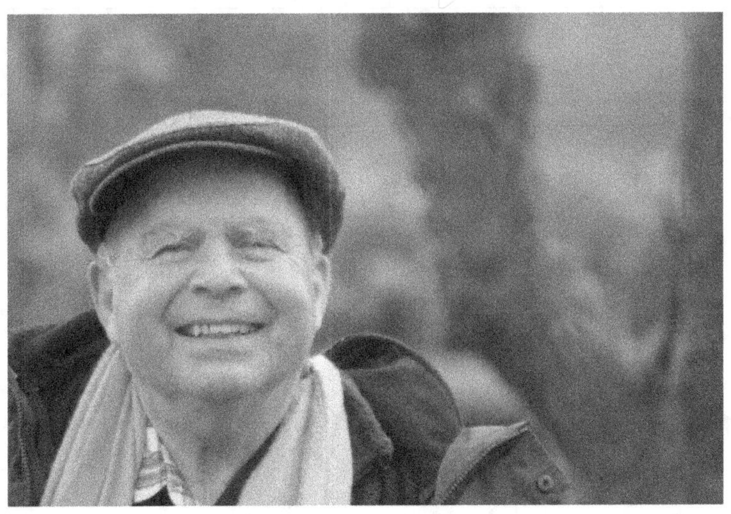

Quercetin	Inhibits RNA polymerase which is necessary for viral replication
Coenzyme Q10	Is necessary for the production of collagen and elastin so keeps tissues supple. It is a strong antioxidant and reduces the risk of blood clots and the rupture of fatty plaques in arteries. Lack of Q10 results in muscle wasting, heart failure, neuropathy and

	injury to tendons and ligaments
Allicin	Allicin can pass through phospholipid membranes of cell and inhibit viral replication even further.
selenium	This is an antiviral which specifically suppresses activity of hemagglutinin and neuraminidase. The former causes blood to clot. It is a glycoprotein which enables fusion between viral and cellular membrane. The latter enable the virus to infect other cells in the host organism. All flu virus have sialic acid which this enzyme cleaves to allow virus to detach from cell.

Please note that bacterial toxins are virulence factors. That is they are weapons that bacteria use to allow them to target host cells function and take over their processes so that microbial infection is able to flourish.

Some toxins directly target innate immune system cells and wipe out the defensive action of the host immune response.

Extra information

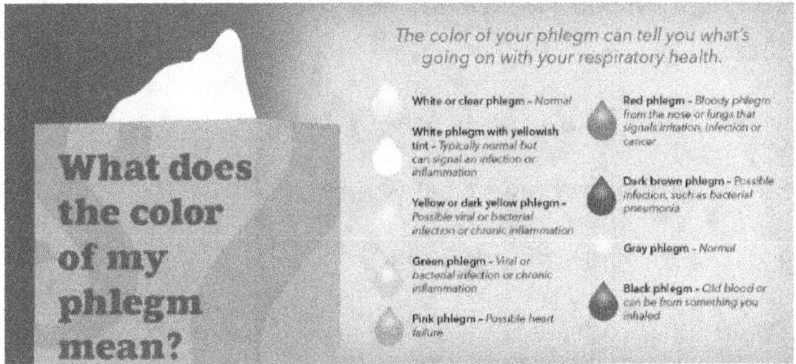

24

Protocol for bronchospasm, thick mucus

The dosage is for daily amounts:

200mcg of selenium (or 2 brazil nuts daily)

N-acetyl cysteine (NAC)[25] – a powerful antioxidant (please not there are various prescribing dosages. Children under two should not be given NAC but there is no harm in increasing foods containing L-Cysteine (see below for the list of common foods.

Children and teenagers can be given 200mg NAC daily

---

[24] https://www.unitypoint.org/news-and-articles/phlegm-cheat-sheet-recognizing-normal-and-concerning-colors-and-consistencies#:~:text=Phlegm%20from%20pneumonia%20can%20be,phlegm%20is%20from%20bacterial%20pneumonia.
[25] NAC is a metabolite – or end product – of cysteine.

Adults normally 600mg in divided doses but up to 900mg in divided doses has been suggested for severe cases.

Magnesium 300mg daily for adults.

65mg for children aged 1-3 years

110 mg for children aged 4-8

300 mg for those above 9 years

High dose vitamin C 2g-4g for adults/teenagers

Children 100mg and upwards until bowel tolerance is reached.

Bowel tolerance may take a while to reach as vitamin C will be used up rapidly.

DMSO (low percent strength) rubbed over the affected parts including sinuses if needed)

Sit in hot steamy bath as humidity helps enormously or breathe in steam from a cup of coffee.

Coffee also helps expel mucus.

Foods containing L-cysteine

Eggs

Poultry

Beef

 Whole grains

Yogurt and cottage cheese

Pork

Chickpeas, legumes, oats

Vegetables from the onion family

Mushrooms

Beef liver